T0273797

MENTAL HEALTH MICROGAINS

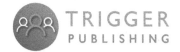

PRAISE FOR *MENTAL HEALTH MICROGAINS*

"You know that much-used phrase, 'Every journey starts with that first step'?

This is a doable, down-to-earth guide, helping you to get to grips with that nagging feeling that, when it comes to your mental health and wellbeing, something is slightly 'off'.

So many of us realize we're feeling flat, low or even struggling, and contentment seems out of grasp.

Let's be clear – nobody 'bounces back'! It's the small, manageable things we tweak that eventually add up to feeling more connected.

Dr Tara and Dr Emma do a fantastic job of giving you the tools to get back on track... step by step."

TRISHA GODDARD, *TV presenter*

ABOUT THE AUTHORS

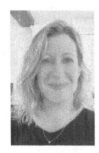

Dr Emma Cotterill is an HCPC Registered Clinical Psychologist with more than 15 years of experience working in the NHS, privately in her own practice, Empower Psychology, and with neuropsychology colleagues at Allied Neuro Therapy. She is dedicated to supporting individuals experiencing mental health difficulties and their families, with specialist experience in exploring issues of grief, loss and trauma. She is passionate about developing thriving mental health and wellbeing for the body and mind. She uses an individualized integrative therapy approach, drawing on CBT, ACT, CFT, EMDR, systemic approaches and mindfulness. Dr Emma is a therapist, writer, supervisor, podcast guest, and trainer, as well as a parent, cat owner, and a music, theatre, fitness and adventure lover.

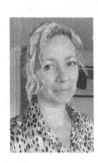

Dr Tara Quinn-Cirillo is an HCPC Registered Counselling Psychologist and Associate Fellow of The British Psychological Society. She has more than 20 years of clinical experience in mental health, neurodivergence, disability and human behaviour. She runs her own private practice in West Sussex, and is the founder and director of The Conversation Starter Project CIC, a grassroots community project tackling emotional health. She is also the founder of the Human Animal Welfare Alliance (HAWA), which supports the emotional health of those working in animal welfare.

Dr Tara is an accomplished broadcaster and media expert globally and the host of *The Adversity Psychologist Podcast*. She has been involved in many innovative collaborations with health and wellbeing platforms, with the aim of bringing high-quality mental health knowledge to the public. Alongside her professional pursuits, she is a parent and owner of two energetic dogs.

MENTAL HEALTH MICROGAINS

50 Small Actions That Will Make a Big Difference to Your Wellbeing

DR EMMA COTTERILL AND
DR TARA QUINN-CIRILLO

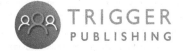

Published in 2024 by Trigger Publishing
An imprint of Shaw Callaghan Ltd

UK Office
The Stanley Building
7 Pancras Square
Kings Cross
London N1C 4AG

US Office
On Point Executive Center, Inc
3030 N Rocky Point Drive W
Suite 150
Tampa, FL 33607
www.triggerpublishing.com

A CIP catalogue record for this book is available upon request from the British Library
ISBN: 978-1-83796-076-7
eBook ISBN: 978-1-83796-077-4

CONTENTS

INTRODUCTION

Taking care of your mental health, learning how to thrive, finding ways to enhance your wellbeing – these are phrases you may be very familiar with.

As a society our knowledge is increasing around the subjects of psychology, mental health and wellbeing. But what does this knowledge mean in practice? How do we break this down into workable, manageable daily steps that will make a real difference to our lives? Let us show you.

Using the concept of "microgains", this book brings you simple ways to take care of your mental health and enhance your wellbeing with small, manageable steps, incorporated into the everyday.

THE CONCEPT OF THE MICROGAIN

Microgains – also known as marginal gains – is a concept developed from the field of sports psychology. It derives from the marginal gains theory (developed by Sir Dave Brailsford), which states that focusing on and making small improvements across a number of areas can lead to a significant overall improvement.

Marginal gains refer to the ability to make small steps, adjustments, changes or improvements, in order to create an overall improvement in performance. These small – or micro – changes may seem minor or subtle, but they can add up to create overall gains that make a big difference.

Brailsford applied this theory to British Cycling when he took over as performance director in 2003, and the resulting outcomes led to a significant improvement in the team's cycling performance and achievement at national and worldwide tournaments (such as the Olympics).[1]

When we apply this concept to enhancing our mental health and wellbeing, we can see how microgains can lead to the build-up of incremental gains, which can result in an overall improvement in our mental health.

What is very important to keep in mind is that each individual microgain is a small part of the bigger picture that will help you thrive. As you read through this book, it may be easy to feel dismissive of a microgain step and think, "It won't make a difference if I try this or not." If you notice yourself doing this, see if you can catch this thought and remind yourself: the idea of mental health microgains is to bring together 50 very small pieces to create a whole. If you introduce these 50 small steps into your life, you will have created an overall holistic approach to your mental health and wellbeing that can create a significant shift toward thriving and living well.

The concept of microgains also enables us to break down wellbeing tasks that might otherwise feel too much or overwhelming. When we think about learning or finding time for a new skill that may benefit us, it can be daunting. Learning and making time for meditation? Moving from being non-active to regularly exercising? Introducing strategies for improving sleep or managing worry? How often does this all feel Just. A. Bit. Too. Much? We may notice thoughts about whether we will be able to do it. We may remember previous attempts when learning or finding time for a new skill was hard, and this may impact how we apply ourselves to a new task. This can lead to avoidance/ putting off the task, or even completely abandoning our goal. However, if we break a task down into small steps (or into a microgain), we can reduce the pressure and overwhelm and are more likely to be able to complete and master the task we are working on.

THE 50 MICROGAINS

We have divided this book into 10 sections, each with five microgains. Each section will explain its core themes and why they're so important to build toward our wellbeing. Each of the five microgains within the section will give you some background and a small challenge to try today.

As you work through the book, you will build a toolkit of 50 microgains to develop as part of your own mental health and wellbeing practices, with the aim of creating lifelong habits.

The 10 sections of this book are:

1. **Mindful Microgains** – Based on the principles of mindfulness to help you practise in daily life
2. **Microgains for Breathing and Grounding** – Gives you the tools to breathe well and ground yourself at times of overwhelm and stress
3. **Compassionate Microgains** – Helps you develop a compassionate voice toward yourself and others
4. **Microgains to Rest and Sleep Well** – Gives you tools to rest more, create balance between work/activity and rest, and sleep well
5. **Social Connection Microgains** – Explores small ways to enhance social connection in your life and the benefits this brings
6. **Movement Microgains** – Explores how movement, exercise and being active can be incorporated into your life
7. **Purposeful Action Microgains** – Gives you five small ways to take useful action in your life to make meaningful change
8. **Microgains to Take Care of Your Emotions** – Provides ways to make sense of and manage your emotions

9. **Microgains for How You Think** – Gives you tools to notice, understand and manage your thinking and your thoughts in effective ways

10. **Microgains About You** – Explores further strategies focused on you

HOW TO USE THIS BOOK

You can use this book in different ways:

- Start at the beginning and work your way through.
- Choose a section that most appeals to you or feels most important to you right now and start there.
- Choose one microgain from each section to start with.

As you work through the microgains, you may find it helpful to:

- Make notes (in the book or in a notebook) on what you are finding helpful, tricky, what has surprised you, or what you want to learn more about.
- Factor in time to practise and gain confidence in using each microgain.

As you begin your microgains practice, all we ask is that you:

- Be curious to learning.
- Be flexible and open to giving something new a try.
- See if you can notice if your mind instantly dismisses something, and ask yourself if it is worth challenging this and being open to it instead.
- Don't give up.

AN IMPORTANT POINT

Hold and apply the ideas in this book lightly and flexibly. Be open to change or adaptation. Avoid "I must" or "I have to" statements; aim instead for "I am choosing to try...".

When we attempt to apply any new ideas/strategies/ practices too intensely or rigidly, they can become unhealthy and dysfunctional. For example, aiming to walk 5,000 steps a day during the week is a potentially feasible healthy task, but pushing yourself to achieve this when you are poorly, have a crisis to attend to, or if you begin to panic or beat yourself up if you don't do it, then it soon becomes unhealthy. So please do be aware of your mindset as you approach these microgains.

CHAPTER 1

MINDFUL MICROGAINS

"Mindfulness is about waking up, connecting with ourselves, and appreciating the fullness of each moment of life. [Jon] Kabat-Zinn calls it, 'The art of conscious living.' It is a profound way to enhance psychological and emotional resilience, and increase life satisfaction"[2]

Russ Harris, psychotherapist

THE MICROGAINS

1. Notice Five Things
2. Perform a Mindful Body Scan
3. Walk Mindfully
4. Try a Simple Meditation
5. Notice the Good

Being mindful means paying attention to your body and mind, your thoughts as they appear, your emotions and physical sensations, and where you are at that moment.

Our minds are great at fast-forwarding to the future, revisiting the past or becoming stuck looking inward, and as we do so, it pulls us out of being fully present in the moment. Mastering the ability to notice and become more aware, at any given moment, of what is going on in our mind and body, with the ability to bring ourselves back to the present world around us, provides us with a useful skill for managing our levels of distress and improving our general emotional and physical health. This skill can also help us manage difficult emotions, thoughts and sensations, including pain (both physical and emotional).

Being mindful helps us to be aware of and respond to our needs, and take care of ourselves more effectively. It supports us to be as present as possible in the "here and now" – for ourselves, our loved ones and our work, and to experience the fullness that life has to offer.

There is a wealth of research highlighting the psychological and physical health benefits of being in the present moment or being "mindfully" in the moment. These include improvements in mood, thinking skills, physical health and relationships.

In these five mindful microgains, we will give you steps to increase your mindful skills, and to become more aware, more present and observing of yourself and the moment you are in.

MICROGAIN 1.1

NOTICE FIVE THINGS

We can spend a lot of time not being "present". Instead, we can be caught up inside our minds, or in our phones/screens. The simple act of bringing ourselves into the present by noticing our surroundings is an essential mindfulness skill we can develop. This can help us be grounded in the moment and can reduce feelings of overwhelm.

This strategy is based on the five senses – noticing what you can *see, hear, touch, taste* and *smell*. You can use this strategy at any time, and without anyone being aware you are practising it – both of which are reasons why it is such a great technique to master. Applying this technique can help bring you firmly into the present and grounded in the here and now (see also Microgain 2.3).

HOW TO NOTICE FIVE THINGS

1. Wherever you are, take some time to sit or stand comfortably. Take a nice, slow breath, in through your nose and out through your mouth.
2. Take a moment to look around you. How often do you take the time to observe and experience your surroundings? Take a moment to notice where you are, and who is around you.
3. Then, notice what you can **see**. Can you fix on one or two things that draw your attention? Consider their shape, colour, any details that you like.
4. What can you **hear**? Any white noise, voices, sounds of nature or industry? Is there anything that is drawing your attention?

5. What can you **touch/feel**? Can you feel the fabric you are wearing, the seat you are on? Is there a breeze, fan or anything else you can feel? Are you warm, or are you cold?
6. What can you **smell**? Are you inside or outside? Are there cooking smells, smells of nature, aromatherapy diffusers, perfumes or anything else you can smell?
7. What can you **taste**? Do you notice any taste or sensation in your mouth?

As you move through these steps, notice how you are able to move your attention to your surroundings and each of your senses and back again. Notice how your attention might be pulled inward to your thoughts, memories, emotions or internal physical sensations as you do this. Notice also how it's possible to move from your internal world of thoughts and feelings back to the five senses and the present moment.

MICROGAIN CHALLENGE

Practise this right now.
Try noticing one thing you can see, hear, touch, taste and smell.

If you find this works well, you can experiment with 5, 4, 3, 2, 1:
5 things you can see, **4** things you can hear, **3** things you can touch, **2** things you can smell and **1** thing you can taste.

Notice what it is like to practise this skill. Notice how present and grounded you feel in the here and now *before and after* doing this.

TOP TIP

Start with a sense that resonates with you. Do you perhaps prefer touch, smell, sounds or even taste? Try choosing one modality/sense to focus on to begin with and gradually build in additional senses from there.

MICROGAIN 1.2

PERFORM A MINDFUL BODY SCAN

A body scan can be a lovely way to connect with your own body and notice how sensations, such as feeling relaxed, happy, anxious, stressed or overwhelmed, may be showing up in the body.

A body scan provides us with a way of monitoring how our bodies are doing; it's a way of slowing down and noticing our physicality in a fast-paced world. We know that our bodies can tell us a lot about how we are doing in our mental health. Stress, sadness, overwhelm, fear, grief, anxiety and anger all have physical manifestations in the body. For example, headaches, tight chest or throat, aches and pains, unsettled stomachs and shallow breathing all give us a clue as to how we are feeling and our mental state. So learning to notice how our feelings may be expressed in the body and what our bodies are carrying are important pieces of the puzzle when looking after our mental health.

During a body scan we aim to draw our attention to how the body feels and particularly how different areas of the body feel. We are supported to literally "scan" different areas of the body from top to bottom, observing any sensations as we go.

THE BODY SCAN

1. Get comfortable. Sit in a cosy chair. Wear comfy clothes if you can. Let your posture be relaxed. Don't put effort into maintaining a certain posture. Begin by focusing on your breathing: rhythmic breathing, slowly in and slowly out. (Whilst these are the ideal conditions, you can do this while sitting or standing, wherever you are, as long as it is safe to do so.)

2. Begin to scan slowly and gently through each part of your body. Key areas can include:
   - Head
   - Jaw
   - Neck
   - Shoulders
   - Back
   - Chest
   - Stomach
   - Hips and pelvis
   - Thighs
   - Lower legs
   - Feet
3. Starting at the top, begin by focusing on your head and see if you are able to notice any sensations you experience or observe there.
4. Take it slowly as you move down through the body. As you move through each part of the body, just slowly breathe and notice what sensations you observe. Press pause as you work from one part of the body to another. Increase the length of pauses each time. Try not to judge any sensations that you observe. Simply notice and name them before moving on to the next part of the body.
5. Take time to end the exercise slowly. Allow yourself time to gently come back into the moment after your body scan. (You might like to use Microgain 1.1 to draw yourself back into the present.)

MICROGAIN CHALLENGE

Take five minutes to try a brief body scan right now.
Start from your head and work down to your toes.

What did it feel like to do this? What sensations did you notice your body carrying? Which parts of the body were feeling relaxed or neutral, and which parts were carrying more tension? How do you think this might connect with how you are feeling?

TOP TIP

Practise the body scan as frequently as you can. Practice makes a big difference to this exercise.

You can also listen to a guided body scan if you prefer to be talked through it (YouTube have a range of these). Some find this stops them rushing through it, ensuring they pause and notice each sensation.

MICROGAIN 1.3

WALK MINDFULLY

Learning how to use mindfulness during an everyday activity such as walking (or hiking, jogging or running) can help us be present and grounded. It gives us an opportunity to bring ourselves clearly into the present, for all the benefits that brings (see page 9).

How often have you taken a walk with your head full of the day's stressors? You may have walked without noticing the route, consumed by the heavy thoughts, memories or feelings weighing down on you. In contrast, how often have you taken a walk where you really noticed the journey, engaged with your senses and returned feeling present and refreshed? The latter is what we hope to achieve in this microgain.

The idea of this mindful walking exercise is to help you really engage in the present moment, physically ground yourself in the action of walking, and bring all your awareness to where you are, how you are and the experience of walking.

HOW TO TAKE A MINDFUL WALK

- Begin your walk (ideally choosing a calming setting amongst nature, but you can do this anywhere – in your local park, along the pavements, etc.).
- Start by gently focusing on your steps. You could gently count up to 10 steps as you walk, and then start again at 1.
- Begin to notice your body, how your feet, heels, legs feel as you walk. Notice your feet landing on the ground, notice the way your legs and arms swing, how your body moves, the position of your arms, neck, shoulders and head.

- Look around you. Take a moment to look at what you can see – notice the details.
- Listen. Notice what you can hear. Notice the sounds, the tone, volume and rhythms.
- Along your walk reach out to touch something – a leaf, a branch, a bench. Notice the feeling, the textures.
- Focus on something you can smell.
- Notice what you can taste.
- Let your mind focus on your senses and the world around you, then move gently back to your body, and the feel and movement of it.

As you walk your mind may naturally be drawn to thoughts, worries, future predictions, memories, past events, judgements and assumptions. This is normal and a natural process your mind takes. Don't be frustrated or critical with yourself if this happens. Notice this. Notice what your mind is saying as if you are an observer, looking in through the window of your mind. Take a moment to notice and name how you feel emotionally and where you feel this in your body. And then gently, just for now, guide yourself back to your mindful walking each time it happens. Draw your attention back to the world around you. Take your time. Allow yourself to be present and just be: walking, noticing, being present in the world around you.

MICROGAIN CHALLENGE

Take at least five minutes for a walking break today.
Follow the steps above for a mindful walk. How does it feel to walk this way? As you become more familiar with this exercise, you can do it for longer.

When you have time, choose a particular walk that you regularly enjoy and practise walking mindfully. Learn to do this regularly.

TOP TIP

Begin with a short walk and build up your time by adding small increments of five minutes. Set a time to walk every day over a period of a week and observe any changes in your walking style or your body over this period, or your ability to bring your attention back to the process of mindful walking, rather than being caught up in your head.

MICROGAIN 1.4

TRY A SIMPLE MEDITATION

One aspect of developing the skill of mindfulness is the ability to meditate. This might be something you are familiar with or something that feels new or alien to you. If it's the latter, stay with us!

This quote about meditation is a helpful myth-busting summary:

"Meditation is not mystical – it's simply a way for us to stop for a moment and be calm. In a busy world, it gives us the permission to pause, breathe and reset."[3]

There are multiple benefits of meditation for our wellbeing and mental health. This microgain is a simple meditation that you can incorporate into your day in five minutes.

Meditation is not a relaxation exercise; it is merely a chance to pause, observe where you are and what is happening in your mind and body, and allow yourself to just be in the moment.

SIMPLE MEDITATION

1. Find a calm space wherever you are.
2. Sit with your back straight in a comfortable position.
3. Bring your attention to your breath and slowly notice its rhythm as you breathe in and out. Just notice the breath as it flows. If you notice your breathing is tight or shallow, you might choose to begin to slow it down and expand the breath a little.

4. Let yourself notice what is going on in your mind. Practise just noticing, like you are looking into your mind as an observer. If you get pulled into any of the thoughts, just gently bring yourself back to the breath. Practise letting yourself notice the thoughts and also letting them come and go. You might notice if your mind is feeling full or racing, or if it is feeling calm and slow paced. *Just notice.*

5. Notice any feeling showing up, or how your body feels.

6. Notice if your mind moves into attending to your senses – what you can see, hear, touch, taste or smell. Gently move it around the senses then back to the breath.

7. Stay here observing for a few minutes, then gently bring yourself back to the present.

MICROGAIN CHALLENGE

Try this exercise for five minutes.

What do you notice? How does it feel? Often meditation can be uncomfortable to start with as we learn to practise observing and noticing. This is normal. Aim to keep practising for five minutes each day.

TOP TIP

As you develop the skill of meditation, see if you can expand the amount of time you meditate or explore a meditation app, such as Headspace or Calm, to create a habit.

MICROGAIN 1.5

NOTICE THE GOOD

GLIMMERS, JOY, GRATITUDE

The human mind has a tendency to focus on the negative – to notice what might go or has gone wrong, to pick up on the worries, the negative thoughts, the problems. It does this as a survival mechanism to identify problems as a way of keeping us safe. It is less primed to notice the good. And yet we know that when we can gently and compassionately allow our minds to notice the good – the joy, the hope, the gratitude, the optimism, the glimmers of light – we can create uplifts in our thoughts and feelings, and boost our overall mental health.

There are different ways we can focus our mind toward the good. This includes:

- Focusing on gratitude – what are you grateful for? This could be anything: being grateful for a person in your life, your job, the roof over your head, your health.
- Focusing on joy – what little moments bring you joy? This could be seeing a sunrise, smelling freshly cut grass, having a hug with a loved one, hearing a favourite song...
- Focusing on the extraordinary on an awe walk. Look around and encourage yourself to see the world in a new light – the sunshine, nature, birdsong, life happening...
- Focusing on what has been good today.
- Focusing on things to be proud of.

- Focusing on what you can do today to move toward your goals.
- Focusing on your strengths.
- Focusing on what you have achieved or the progress you have made.
- Focusing on glimmers. "Glimmers" is a term used to describe the opposite of things that trigger us – light, love, things that calm and soothe us, and help us feel at peace.
- Focusing on positive affirmations when you speak to yourself (Microgain 3.2).
- Focusing on an optimistic mindset for your day – e.g., "Today will be a good day".

Read through this list and see if you can notice how many of these (if any) you think you naturally do, or not! Reflect on how it might feel to be able to introduce more of these into your daily habits.

MICROGAIN CHALLENGE

Choose one of the list items above.

Write down three things about yourself, your day or your life that connect to the item you have chosen. Allow yourself to reflect on the words you use, let yourself notice the good and sit with that; see how it feels.

Make a commitment to yourself that for 30 seconds each day this week, you will pause to notice the good.

TOP TIP

Consider starting a journal as a focal point for your reflections. Try and write in this every day. Choose a set time each day to journal – this will help it become a routine activity.

CHAPTER 2

MICROGAINS FOR BREATHING AND GROUNDING

"What has to be taught first, is the breath." [4]

Confucius, philosopher

"Feelings come and go like clouds in a windy sky, conscious breathing is my anchor." [5]

Thich Nhat Hanh, Buddhist monk

THE MICROGAINS

1. Take a Deep Breath
2. Try a Simple Breathing Exercise
3. Ground Yourself When You're Overwhelmed
4. Find Quick Ways to Ground Yourself
5. Create a Calm Space

Being able to breathe well is a powerful tool we can use any time, anywhere. Taking slow, deep breaths has been found to help calm, soothe and regulate the nervous system, helping us move from sympathetic nervous system activation (our fight-or-flight response) to a parasympathetic nervous system activation (our rest-and-digest system).

Conscious breathing – being able to breathe with intention – is something we can learn to do in a few simple steps. With regular practice we can become very familiar with the feelings this state of breathing brings – versus, for example, tense breathing during times of anxiety, stress or overwhelm. Learning how to breathe is a tool we can then use to help calm ourselves and helps us regulate our emotions in challenging times.

Please bear with us for this section! It may sound cliché or obvious (even patronizing) to tell you to "just take a deep breath"; but many of us have never actually been taught how to breathe well and deeply.

Deep breathing on its own doesn't necessarily solve how you are feeling – just like any of these microgains individually won't automatically make miracle changes to your mental health – but once you have developed this skill, you can add it to your repertoire as one small way (microgain!) to help support your wellbeing.

Alongside our tools of deep, conscious, intentional, slow breathing is the ability to ground or anchor ourselves in the moment. This is our ability to physically and mentally ground ourselves, to connect the body and mind to our senses and the world around us, to help us stay strong, stable and anchored through any emotional storm. This is a simple strategy to add to your toolkit for use in stressful times.

MICROGAIN 2.1

TAKE A DEEP BREATH

Learning how to breathe well is a powerful skill we can all develop. It is very common, especially during times of stress, anxiety or overwhelm, for breathing to become shallow or restricted. Sometimes we notice this (e.g., during moments of heightened panic), but at other times, changes to our breathing can happen gradually without us being aware, and can create a chronic pattern of restricted/shallow breathing. This can have a negative impact on our nervous systems, mental health and how we feel physically.

A simple but effective technique we can learn is abdominal or belly breathing. This is a method for taking a slow, deep breath, and can be used to calm overwhelm, and promote clear thinking and decision making.

So let's start.

BELLY BREATHING

- Sit up comfortably in a chair where you feel well supported. (If you can't sit, you can also do this standing in a comfortable position with both feet on the floor, or even lying flat and comfortably in bed or on the sofa.)
- Place your dominant hand (writing hand) on your lower abdomen (your tummy). Place your other hand across your chest so your thumb and pointer finger are running along your collarbone.
- Take a moment to monitor (just notice) your breathing without changing anything. Do you breathe from your chest or your belly? Which hand moves more? How slow or quick does

your breathing feel naturally? Most people will find they are "chest" breathers (mostly breathing from up in your chest). However, if you are someone who does Pilates/yoga, or you have practised deep breathing before, you may have developed belly breathing as your breathing style.

- Take a long, slow in-breath through your nose, and watch as your lower abdomen (tummy) rises like a beachball or like you are blowing up a balloon. Watch it rise/"inflate" (push out/fill up) as you slowly *breathe in* and notice the hand resting on your tummy rising. As you do this, your lungs are filling up from the very bottom. You might also notice your sides, and even your back, begin to expand outwardly as the lungs inflate from all sides.

- Start with breathing in for a slow count of three. As you practise this, see if you can breathe in longer and deeper, for counts of 3, 4, 5...

- As you reach the top of the in-breath, hold the breath for a moment or two, then slowly release the breath back out through your mouth, like you are blowing through a straw. Again, you might start with breathing out for three, but as you practise, see if you can make the out-breath slower and longer, even longer than the in-breath if you can, for 3, 4, 5, 6, 7, 8...

- As you slowly breathe in and out, it can also help to pay attention to your hands. Can you feel the hand on your tummy rise and fall as you breathe? And can you keep the hand on your chest as still as possible? Keeping the hand on your chest still helps you to reduce shallow/chest/restricted breathing, and allows you to move closer to belly breathing. As you begin to master this technique, you will notice that your hand on your chest will remain more and more still.

MICROGAIN CHALLENGE

Practise this exercise for one minute.

Notice how this feels. Can you set a plan to practise this each day? For example, when you are lying in bed, waiting for the kettle to boil or sitting at your desk before you start the day?

TOP TIP

If you are struggling to get a deep in-breath, start with the out-breath. Slowly and gently blow all the air out of your lungs first, then focus on the slow, deep breath in.

MICROGAIN 2.2

TRY A SIMPLE BREATHING EXERCISE

If you've tried Microgain 2.1, you know how a deep breath feels. Now we are going to try experimenting with some variation on this exercise so you can find your favourite. Try each exercise here and see how they feel. It's important to find a way to breathe deeply with which you connect, and which feels calming and soothing.

Initially, try and practise these exercises when you are not anxious, stressed or overwhelmed – for example, when you're lying in bed in the morning, or when having your morning cuppa. This helps you to master the technique so you can effectively apply it at times of stress.

Before you try the below exercises, make sure you have worked through Microgain 2.1 and practised the technical elements of how to take a deep breath.

COLOUR BREATH

- Take a slow, deep breath in through your nose.
- As you breathe in, imagine a soothing, calming colour washing through you.
- Pause for a moment, holding the breath.
- Slowly breathe out, either through your nose or mouth (whichever is more comfortable).

- As you breathe out, imagine breathing out stress and tension, giving this a colour, and imagine that colour leaving you with the out-breath.
- Repeat three times.

CALMING WORD BREATH

- Take a slow, deep breath in through your nose.
- As you breathe in, imagine a soothing, calming word or phrase that you can say to yourself – e.g., "Calm"; "Peace"; "Rest"; "I'm okay"; "I'm safe"; "I can get through this"; "This is tough, but I can do this".
- Pause for a moment, holding the breath.
- Slowly breathe out through your nose or mouth, saying this word or phrase in your mind.
- Repeat three times.

4 X 4 BREATHING

Picture a square. Imagine tracing along the sides of the square with each of the steps below, starting in the bottom left corner.

- Take a slow, deep breath in through your nose for a count of four (imagine tracing up the left side of the square).
- Gently hold the breath for four counts (trace along the top of the square).
- Slowly breathe out through your nose or mouth for four counts (trace down the right side of the square).
- Hold the breath for four counts (trace along the bottom of the square).
- Repeat three times.

MOVEMENT AND BREATHING

- Place your hands together in front of you.
- Take a slow, deep breath in through your nose.
- As you breathe in, stretch your arms out wide to the sides.
- Pause for a moment, holding the breath.
- Slowly breathe out through your nose or mouth, and as you do, slowly bring your hands and arms gently back in front of you.
- Repeat this three times.

MICROGAIN CHALLENGE

Choose one or more of the exercises in this microgain to gently practise now.

Make a note of how each exercise feels. Schedule a time each day to practise. Keep it simple – just three breaths, 30 seconds of your time.

TOP TIP

As you pause and hold the breath, really notice the feeling of slowing down, calming body and mind.

MICROGAIN 2.3

GROUND YOURSELF WHEN YOU'RE OVERWHELMED

GROUNDING/DROPPING THE ANCHOR

This microgain technique is useful for helping you become grounded in the moment – at a time when you may feel overwhelmed in a difficult situation or with difficult thoughts, feelings or physical sensations.

When the nervous system is in threat mode, when our bodies are carrying lots of stress, or when we're feeling intense emotions, racing thoughts or strong physical sensations, it can be helpful to have a strategy that can ground or anchor us.

The "drop the anchor" technique, used often by Russ Harris, relates to the imagery of a ship that is adrift at sea or in the midst of a storm (representing how we may feel when we are overwhelmed or in the middle of an "emotional storm"). By "dropping the anchor", the ship will stay in one place in the midst of the unsettled storm, and stay contained and stable until the storm has passed. (Russ provides free audio resources for practising this technique on his website. See the Resources list at the back of the book.) This is what we want to achieve for ourselves with this approach.

If we learn skills to become more grounded in the moment, we can then learn to:

• Hold ourselves steady and feel able to cope in the midst of a challenging experience

- Better observe what is happening for us in the moment
- Decide how to respond to what we notice
- Stay in a calm place until the crisis /challenging experience has passed

HOW TO GROUND YOURSELF

- Sit upright or stand somewhere comfortable, where you feel well supported.
- Take an in-breath through your nose for about three seconds. Breathe out slowly to the count of three.
- Gently push your feet into the floor. Imagine you are dropping an anchor and grounding yourself in the here and now, holding yourself steady. Observe the sensation of physically connecting to the ground as you do so. If you are sitting on a chair, you may *gently* push your bottom back in the seat, or your back against the back of the chair. (Note: This exercise is about making contact with the physical world around you and observing the grounding sensations. It should not feel uncomfortable or painful.)
- Gently press your hands together – either in a templed position or clasping your hands together – and lightly apply pressure (again, so that you can feel this but not so it is uncomfortable).
- Spend a few moments noticing your internal world. Are there any emotions, thoughts or other physical sensations you observe? Notice and name them to yourself. Just notice and name; don't engage with them. Don't try to push them away. For example: "I am feeling very stressed – I can feel this in my chest. I can notice my mind racing with thoughts about the situation."
- Gently move your attention wider.

- Notice your body, how it is feeling, and the sense of it becoming anchored and grounded. (Again, gently notice the feeling of your hands pushing together and your feet pushing into the floor.)
- Now have a little look around the room you are in. Notice and name something you can see, hear, touch, taste or smell.
- Slowly breathe. Notice you are in this moment, right here, right now. You are experiencing this emotional storm. And you are anchored and steady in the midst of the storm.
- Stay in this state for another minute, or as long as you feel you need.

How do you feel after grounding compared to when you started?

MICROGAIN CHALLENGE

Try this grounding/dropping-anchor technique today.

Try this exercise for between 1–5 minutes, depending on how you are feeling, aiming to bring the exercise to a close as you feel grounded and anchored. Imagine dropping the anchor in the storm, or being an oak tree with deep, strong roots, and hold yourself gently grounded until you notice the storm begin to abate.

TOP TIP

When you begin to practise dropping anchor, do this when you are not in an anxious/stressed/overwhelmed state. This will help you focus and remember the process of the exercise when you need to use it in times of stress.

MICROGAIN 2.4

FIND QUICK WAYS TO GROUND YOURSELF

As we've learned so far, grounding can positively impact our health and wellbeing by improving sleep and stress levels, and soothing us. There are many wonderful ways to ground ourselves when we feel overwhelmed. You can experiment with what works for you. Build up a little toolkit of grounding techniques unique to your needs on different days.

Building from Microgain 2.3, some additional or alternative ways to ground yourself include the following.

SCENT

Smell is a powerful tool for grounding. Smells have the ability to instantly bring us back to the present moment. You can use vaporizers, aromatherapy sprays, roll-on sticks (lavender is a favourite calming smell), perfumes or flowers to gently smell or spray in the air around you.

FEET ON GRASS

A really lovely grounding exercise is to place your bare feet directly on grass. Feel the soles of your feet as they make contact with the grass. Gently wriggle your toes and pay attention to the sensation. You can also do this with a carpet or textured rug, or when walking on sand or along the seashore.

FRESH AIR

Stand outside and allow yourself to feel the air – the warmth or cold, the wind or rain on your face. Give yourself a moment to feel connected to the world around you.

WARMTH

Gentle warmth can also be an effective grounding method. Try gentle warmth in the mouth – drink a hot beverage and hold the liquid in your mouth for a few moments before swallowing. Or try placing your hands in warm water or using a hand warmer.

COLD

The body responds to sudden intense coldness by shifting its physiological response. This often reduces the adrenalin you may be feeling. Using the cold to ground yourself can help when you feel intense emotions such as anxiety – the cold helps to bring you back to the here and now, and calm or slow the impact of your emotions. (Note: If you are new to using cool temperatures to ground, slowly build up the intensity of the temperature.) Here are few ideas:

- Place your hands in a sink of tepid water for a few moments. You can slowly add colder water to see what this feels like for you. Build up the intensity by running only the cold tap and then adding a couple of ice cubes to the water. As you become accustomed to this technique, you can try filling the sink with ice and water and splashing your face.
- Hold an ice cube in your hand for a few moments. To protect your skin, use a thin cloth around the ice cube.

- Slowly drink ice-cold water from a glass. Pay attention to how the water feels as it is in your mouth and as it runs down your throat.

PHYSICAL MOVEMENT

Moving your body and making slow and considered movements is a great way to ground yourself. Try making circular movements with your arms or rotating your hips in a circular motion. Using dance moves can also be a fun way to make exaggerated movements with your arms, hips and legs.

MICROGAIN CHALLENGE

Choose one grounding technique from the options above.

Try this for five minutes. What do you notice in your body as you immerse yourself in that particular grounding exercise? What happens to your emotions? Do they become less dominant or intense?

TOP TIP

It can take time to master grounding techniques. We may not notice an immediate reduction in our emotions or thought patterns. This is normal. Remember, we are not trying to get rid of difficult emotions or stresses, only to help ourselves be more able to manage and respond to them.

MICROGAIN 2.5

CREATE A CALM SPACE

Imagine a calm space that helps you feel safe and soothed. Being in a serene, safe space can diffuse intense feelings by calming the nervous system and reducing the sense of threat – it can also facilitate a calmer lifestyle. By purposefully creating safe spaces in the everyday, we can enhance our ability to nurture ourselves and build up resilience to life's demands.

This calm, safe space can be something in real life/the physical world, or something we create in our minds. Both can be equally useful.

IN REAL LIFE

A calm, safe space in real life could be created in a bedroom, office or garden space. This might also take the form of a space you have access to in the immediate world around you, for example, a nature spot, by water or other local beauty spot.

To set up a place like this of your own, you can:

- Create a calm space in a room, or within a room, such as a corner of your living room. This is a good option if you've got limited space or you're living with family.
- Create a portable calm space – e.g., set up your bathroom for a warm sensory bath, create some space when travelling to journal and pause.
- Create an outside calm space in a garden.

When creating a calm, safe space, consider:

- Light levels
- Colours
- Textures and fabrics
- Noise – such as soothing music, white noise, nature sounds
- Reducing clutter
- Temperature
- Scents

IN YOUR IMAGINATION

A familiar exercise in therapy is to create a calming, safe space in your imagination. To do this:

- Start by choosing a space you can go in your mind that feels calm or safe. This might be a place you have been in real life or an entirely imaginary space. It might be by the sea, a river, in the woods, on the beach, a mountain or in a city – anywhere that feels calm or safe to you.
- Once you have found "your place", then build up the image of your space by imagining the following:
  - What you can see
  - What you can hear
  - What you can touch, taste or smell
  - What the temperature is like, or the weather
  - What the light is like
- In a quiet space, take a moment to close your eyes and immerse yourself in this imaginary image. Really feel the senses and what it would be like in your space. Let yourself know that this is your space to come to in your imagination, any time you need to feel calm, safe and soothed.

The benefit of an imaginary space is that we can close your eyes and conjure it any time, anywhere (lying in bed, on the bus, in a dentist's waiting room, before going into a meeting, etc.).

MICROGAIN CHALLENGE

Think about where you can begin to create a calm space in your life, both in reality and in your imagination. Focus on building up one of these areas today.

TOP TIP

Creating a space in reality isn't solely about practical elements and doesn't have to involve cost. Think about how you can personalize the space with what you have available. How can you create more natural light? What things do you already have that make you feel calm, that have meaning for you and elicit calm memories? These can be objects, pictures or photographs – anything that helps soothe you.

CHAPTER 3

COMPASSIONATE MICROGAINS

"Our human compassion binds us the one to the other – not in pity or patronizingly, but as human beings who have learnt how to turn our common suffering into hope for the future."[6]

President Nelson Mandela

THE MICROGAINS

1. Be Self-Compassionate
2. Recite Compassionate Affirmations
3. Use Compassionate Touch
4. Show Compassion for Others
5. Harness the Power of AND

To be compassionate to ourselves and others is a wonderful human quality. It is also one that many of us find difficult to do. We perhaps find it easier (although not always) to extend compassion to others, but we can often find it very difficult to extend that compassion to ourselves. Too often, instead, we use a critical, harsh inner voice.

Compassion can be seen in how we speak to ourselves, in how we behave toward ourselves and how we extend compassion to others. Compassion is about showing kindness, understanding and support in the face of challenges. Being compassionate benefits our mental health in many ways. People who are compassionate are able to experience benefits in mood and flexibility of thinking, have a growth mindset, be more forgiving and resilient, and work more effectively toward their goals.

MICROGAIN 3.1

BE SELF-COMPASSIONATE

How do you speak to yourself? Are you kind or critical? Supportive or judgemental?

Self-compassion is the ability to be compassionate to ourselves – both during our day-to-day lives and when we find ourselves in challenging situations. Being compassionate to ourselves is an alternative to the critical, judgemental or harsh inner voice that many of us carry inside, or have learnt to apply to ourselves.

Self-compassion researcher Kristin Neff has identified three principles of self-compassion:

- **Mindfulness** – the ability to step back and see the situation fairly, compassionately and non-judgementally. Neff talks about the idea of "neither suppressing or exaggerating" the challenges or situations we may find ourselves in.
- **Common humanity** – the idea that we are only human, and we are not infallible. We are not alone in making mistakes, failures, being flawed, being overwhelmed and so on. Holding this idea in mind is an essential part of enabling us to hold self-compassion for ourselves.
- **Self-kindness** – being kind and understanding of ourselves and the situations we find ourselves in. It means we are empathic and gentle on ourselves, as we would be with a friend, child or loved one.[7]

Importantly (and this is a common fear of those unsure about practising self-compassion), self-compassion is not "letting ourselves off the hook". It is kindly, fairy, firmly and compassionately acknowledging the situations we may be in and considering the whole context in which we find ourselves – the idea of compassionately considering what we have gone through, rather than what is wrong with us. A compassionate voice allows us to be understanding and kind to ourselves, AND also acknowledges (kindly) where we may have made errors or could do things differently, and helps us focus on how to do this.

A compassionate approach is beneficial for our mental health in multiple ways. It is connected to improved mood and optimism, self-worth and body satisfaction; increased levels of resilience, motivation and determination; and improved boundaries, connection and work-life balance. Interestingly, it also enables us to achieve – people who are self-critical often think they need this critical voice (rather than a compassionate one) to achieve their goals, but this is simply not true!

MICROGAIN CHALLENGE

Think of a situation where you felt cross, unkind or critical toward yourself.

- Choose something that is around a 5 out of 10 in terms of difficulty or frustration for this exercise. Maybe you forgot to pack your child something they needed for school, or you made a mistake in your work, or you missed your turn when driving.
- Consider how you have been talking to yourself about this situation and how you could make this more compassionate. If you are stuck, remember Neff's self-compassion principles.[8] Try a version of:

This situation was tough/stressful/difficult.

I am only human; I'm not alone in struggling with this/making this mistake.

I can forgive myself/be kind to myself/understand what was going on for me that contributed to this happening.

Notice how it feels to practise using a more self-compassionate voice.

Can you find one moment to practise using a self-compassionate voice today instead of a critical one?

TOP TIP

Try imagining how you would talk to a friend in the same situation. How would you speak to them if you were being compassionate? What words could you use? What would happen if you used these same compassionate words on yourself?

MICROGAIN 3.2

RECITE COMPASSIONATE AFFIRMATIONS

In psychology and neuropsychology, we often talk about neuroplasticity. This term describes the brain's ability to adapt and change to the environment around it. Essentially, the neural pathways in the brain can change through growth and reorganization.

Neuroplasticity can be impacted by our experiences, the way we think and the way we behave. When this happens the brain can function in a way different to before. One neuroplasticity exercise is to begin to use positive affirmations to positively impact the way that we think about ourselves and our abilities. When we do this we begin to reinforce the neural pathways that can focus on positive thinking over negative thinking.

Affirmation is a useful concept to provide emotional or supportive encouragement to ourselves. We can use affirmations to help us navigate difficult events or to give us motivation when we need it or are a little "stuck".

Affirmations consist of phrases with a positive element to help us feel hopeful and confident about our current situations – for example, when we have specific, tough tasks to do; when we face difficult times; or simply when we need to shape our focus and mindsets at the beginning of the day.

If we gently bring in affirmations as part of our daily routines, we can begin to change the way that we think and ultimately view ourselves.

POSITIVE AFFIRMATIONS EXAMPLES

Personal statements

- I am good enough.
- I can do X or Y.
- I love being me.
- I have a lot to offer.
- I have potential.
- I am capable.
- I am loving.
- I can overcome adversity.
- I can inspire others.
- I am doing the best I can.
- I deserve happiness.
- I can try new things.
- I am grateful.
- I can be compassionate to myself.
- Difficult times will pass.

Skill development

- It is OK to look after myself.
- I matter.
- I am learning to do X really well.
- I am trying.
- I am improving my physical health.

HOW TO INCORPORATE AFFIRMATIONS INTO YOUR DAILY LIFE

- Make a list of your own favourite/personal affirmations.
- Say your affirmations out loud – try walking around saying them.

- Write down your top three affirmations in your phone or diary where you can read them each day.
- Record some affirmations on a voice memo and play them back at regular intervals.
- Write affirmations on Post-it notes and place these around your home.
- Choose some songs to add to your playlist that fit with your affirmations.
- Use your affirmations as journaling prompts to inspire you to really engage with the affirmation and what it means for you.
- Use your top three affirmations combined with the kind hands exercise (Microgain 3.3).
- Choose set times of day to purposefully repeat affirmations to yourself, such as when you get ready in the morning and look in the mirror, or when you get in the car to drive home from work.

MICROGAIN CHALLENGE

Choose your top three affirmations from the list above, or develop your own.

Write these down somewhere you can check back on them easily at any time. Say them slowly to yourself now, and allow yourself to really feel the meaning of each affirmation in your mind and body. Each morning this week, take a quiet moment for yourself to repeat the affirmations.

TOP TIP

Try looking in the mirror when practising your affirmations. You may feel self-conscious at first, but this will help you connect with yourself.

MICROGAIN 3.3

USE COMPASSIONATE TOUCH

A simple exercise we can do at any time to bring compassionate soothing into our mind and body is the soothing touch, or kind hands, exercise, which is developed and adapted from the work of Kristin Neff and Russ Harris. (See the Resources at the back of the book for more information.)

Using compassionate touch is beneficial because this creates physical touch and warmth, which stimulates oxytocin production (known as the "love hormone" that promotes positive feelings in our minds and bodies), and activates the parasympathetic (our in-built self-soothing) system. This is the system that is activated when newborn babies are placed skin to skin on their caregiver.

The process of compassionate physical touch slows down breathing, heart rate and blood pressure, and calms the nervous system, making us feel relaxed. We can activate the parasympathetic system at any time with this exercise, which means we can use it whenever and wherever we are.

SOOTHING TOUCH AND KIND HANDS EXERCISE

You can do these anywhere with only a minute or two to spare. You can do these when you are feeling calm, and you can do these at times of stress or suffering.

Soothing touch
- Sit comfortably in a chair or stand.
- Gently breathe in through your nose and out through your mouth.

- Softly place your dominant hand skin to skin along your opposite collarbone, so if you are right-handed, place your right hand on your left collarbone.
- Feel the skin-to-skin contact. Notice how your body feels.
- Gently place your other hand on top of the hand that is already touching your collarbone and chest. Push your arms gently in at your sides. Feel the supportive touch.
- Continue to breathe in and out gently.
- Continue this for as long as you need.
- Notice how your body feels, how soothed it feels.

Kind hands

- Take a slow, deep breath.
- Reach your hand out and turn it, holding it palm up.
- Take a moment to think about your hand and visualize all the kind things your hand has done (e.g., stroked a pet, held your partner's hand, cuddled your child, stroked a loved one's hair...). Imagine all this kindness in the palm of your hand.
- Place your hand on your heart, or on the part of your body where you feel any emotional discomfort or stress (this can be over your clothes, or skin to skin).
- Notice the warmth radiating from your hand into your body.
- Imagine this warmth radiating inward, around the parts of your body which are feeling stress, discomfort, pain or tension.
- Imagine this warmth as gentle, kind, soothing, compassionate feelings that you are sending to yourself.
- Add a kind word if you would like, such as "You are okay", "You can do this", "This is tough", "You can get through this", "Take your time", "Just breathe".
- Take a moment to send and receive this warmth and kindness.

WHEN YOU CAN USE THESE EXERCISES

- First thing in the morning
- Last thing at night
- When you are feeling sad, anxious or stressed
- When you notice you are holding physical tension in your body
- Before you are about to do something tough, or you have just experienced something distressing

MICROGAIN CHALLENGE

Practise one of these exercises for one minute today.

Notice how it feels and how your body and mind respond. Build this into your daily routine – for example, once in the morning and once in the evening before bed, or any other time you notice you need care.

TOP TIP

Gently warm your hands before placing them skin to skin for increased benefit.

MICROGAIN 3.4

SHOW COMPASSION FOR OTHERS

Compassion can be beneficial not only in how we treat ourselves, but how we relate to others as well. So often in recent years, we hear people state on social media that we should all "be kind". This is a wonderful sentiment, but one that people sometimes struggle to implement.

Extending our compassion for others means – in the same way that we are learning to do for ourselves – that we maintain a compassionate stance, and hold in mind that others are only human too; they are fallible, flawed, prone to mistakes and not always acting wisely. It means holding in mind the bigger picture of what might be going on for a person and why they may have made the decisions (or mistakes) they did. It means holding people responsible for their actions, but doing so gently, compassionately, and with empathy and forgiveness.

Compassion for others can improve our wellbeing by helping us reduce any anger, resentments, hostility, dislike, judgement or criticism we may be holding toward others. It enables us to feel more warmth and compassion, and feel at peace rather than holding on to negative feelings. We can hold compassion whilst also maintaining boundaries around how much we let people be part of our lives.

PRACTISING COMPASSION

There are times when you can practise compassion for others in small ways – for example:

- When a mistake is made
- When someone cancels at short notice or is late

- When someone is irritable or snappy with you
- When someone knocks or rushes past you
- When someone doesn't message you back
- When a colleague doesn't complete a task you are working on jointly
- When someone falls in front of you
- When a friend messages too frequently during a stressful time
- When a neighbour becomes reliant on you during a tough time

We can practise or show compassion for others in many ways – for example:

- Ask: "How can I view this through the most compassionate lens possible?"
- Consider times when you have exhibited the same behaviour and how you might understand this in yourself (if you are compassionate toward yourself!); or imagine this was a dear friend/loved one/child.
- Be curious to consider or understand compassionately what might be going on for a person for this behaviour to happen.
- Remind yourself that we are only human, we all make mistakes and can be flawed, whilst still being good people.
- Be open to listening to what is going on for a person. Take time to hear – really hear – when they speak to you. In a fast-paced world, we may not really take the time to listen to their experiences and needs.
- Show care with your tone and body language. This is a free and underrated way of making people see you care.
- Carve out or allocate time to spend with family or friends. We can often forget to have quality time with those who are special to us. It can help us connect with them and their needs.
- Be patient, accepting and forgiving.

MICROGAIN CHALLENGE

Consider a situation where someone has annoyed or irritated you or you felt yourself forming a negative opinion about them.
This could be someone in your life, or someone you have seen or read about in the media. Go through the compassionate practices above for the individual you have in mind, and see if you can allow yourself to soften and find compassion for this person and the situation they may find themselves in.

TOP TIP

Identify someone in your life to practise compassion with. Don't feel you have to apply this to everyone in your life at the same time. Start small and build up from there. Start with some simple steps, such as listening to someone or checking in with them. Be open, honest and empathetic.

MICROGAIN 3.5

HARNESS THE POWER OF AND

A simple and compassionate tool we can use every day is the word AND.

Too often we can form judgements, conclusions and narratives about ourselves and others that end up focusing on only one thing or one aspect of a situation. For example: "I'm sad", "This is too hard", "That behaviour is terrible".

When we focus only on one aspect of a situation or feeling, this often closes down or narrows our perspective and makes it hard to hold a wider, or more human, compassionate perspective.

The power of AND is such a simple concept that we can apply to any situation. By adding in the word AND, we open up the way we understand a situation, ourselves or others. It makes room for more possibilities, more hope and more compassion.

The power of AND also helps remind us that we are all only human and we can experience two or more things at one time. We are not one unitary thing – we can feel different things at once; we can have multiple intentions at once. This idea brings in compassion for ourselves and others.

HOW TO USE THE POWER OF AND

Consider these statements:

- I can be sad AND grateful.
- I can be angry AND hurting.
- I can be overwhelmed AND hopeful.
- I can be scared AND brave.

- I can be furious AND still care.
- This is hard, AND I can find a way through.
- That behaviour might be not OK, AND I can acknowledge they are only human.
- They have hurt me, AND I know they care for me/didn't do it intentionally.
- This situation is devastating, AND I can find moments of joy.
- I can be understanding AND keep my boundaries.

MICROGAIN CHALLENGE

Make a note on your phone/in a diary or notebook to remind yourself of the power of AND.

As you go through your day, see if you can add in the word AND when you are describing yourself, others or a situation, to help widen out your perspective and bring more hope and compassion to the situation.

TOP TIP

Start small for issues that bother you only in small ways and see if you can add an AND in. For example:

- I am feeling tired AND I am excited to go out tonight.
- The journey to work was stressful, AND I can focus on making the best of the rest of the day.
- I missed my alarm AND I can prioritize what I need to do and leave the rest.

CHAPTER 4

MICROGAINS TO REST AND SLEEP WELL

"Wisdom is knowing when to have rest, when to have activity, and how much of each to have."[9]

Sri Sri Ravi Shankar, yoga teacher and spiritual leader

"Do but consider what an excellent thing sleep is... that golden chain that ties health and our bodies together."[10]

Thomas Dekker, writer

THE MICROGAINS

1. Slow Down, Press Pause, Find Balance
2. Rest Well
3. Improve Your Sleep Routine
4. Get to (or Back to) Sleep
5. Reduce Alcohol and Caffeine

How we rest and how we sleep make such a difference to our lives. Yet we so often disregard or don't get round to prioritizing this.

Rest is something we can engage in throughout our day, ensuring there is a balance of rest amongst work and activity. Rest, of course, encompasses sleep, but it also includes how we spend our time in the day. Good and productive rest is restorative – it restores our energy. It enables us to be more productive and more effective in our daily activities.

Often, we can find ourselves resting only once we become exhausted, burnt out or worn out. However, this is often less helpful than if we had rested BEFORE this process. Valuing rest as a crucial part of our self-care and wellbeing routine helps prevent us reaching exhaustion and burnout, and enables us to stay well in the long run.

One part of rest is our time spent sleeping, and this is, as most of us know, an essential part of our wellbeing and mental health. Sleeping well impacts everything from mood, energy levels, metabolism, digestion and physical health, to motivation, memory, decision-making abilities and so much more. Creating sleep habits and successful sleep strategies can benefit you in many ways.

MICROGAIN 4.1

SLOW DOWN, PRESS PAUSE, FIND BALANCE

We live in a fast-paced world. Our lives are full. Full of work, admin, chores, parenting, caring, exercising, learning, training, commuting and socializing. And alongside this is a never-ending stream of information coming from our phones, screens, laptops and tablets. We are also living in an "immediate" world – deliveries can come the next day; takeaways can be on our doorsteps in 30 minutes; if we want to know something, we can look it up instantly. Whether we fully realize it or not, our pace of life is busy, constant and pressured. So within this fast pace, finding time to slow down can be incredibly beneficial, but it can also can feel alien to us, when everything around us is busy.

Creating a slower pace in our minds and bodies, even for a few moments, can help bring a sense of soothing and calm, and a chance to de-stress.

HOW TO PRESS PAUSE

Consider the following for micro-ways to create a moment to slow down in your day:

- Delay looking at your phone for 30 minutes to one hour after waking.
- Start your day, as you lie in bed, with a breathing exercise (Microgain 2.2), gratitude practice (Microgain 1.5) or meditation (Microgain 1.4).

- Perform a slow yoga stretch (Microgain 6.2).
- Take your time as you brush your hair or put on your moisturizer – imagine you are in a salon, using slow, soothing, relaxing movements.
- Slow down your pace as you walk.
- Use your breathing exercises at multiple times in the day – try them while waiting for the kettle to boil, on the train or in a meeting...
- Avoid multi-tasking – do one thing at a time.
- Sit in the garden or in a comfortable space whilst you enjoy a tea of coffee break, even for a few minutes.
- Give yourself five minutes in nature – just to pause and listen, taking in all the senses.
- Delegate a task so you have one less thing to do today.
- Push back your schedule/plans/expectations so you can give yourself permission to have more rest and less "doing" time.
- Allow more time between activities to prevent rushing.
- Make a note to tackle a task, but don't do it immediately – let it wait.
- Mindfully make a hot drink, and take your time to sit and savour the flavour and warmth.

MICROGAIN CHALLENGE

Choose one way you can slow down today – from the list above or your own ideas.

As you try this, notice how it feels to slow down, to do less, to rest, to breathe, to take time for yourself.

TOP TIP

A useful way to introduce the concept of pressing pause in your day is to try saying "pause" out loud to yourself during different times of the day. Imagine pressing a button on a remote control that pauses you in the moment. Simply sit, pause, breathe and observe.

MICROGAIN 4.2

REST WELL

GIVE YOURSELF PERMISSION TO REST

Rest is one of the most important things we can do for ourselves, and often the thing we least give ourselves. Unhelpful ideas, such as needing to earn our rest, often unconsciously influence our thinking and behaviour. Only choosing rest when we are exhausted is another. We might struggle to know how to rest, or we may not even believe that it is okay to rest. Perhaps rest feels lazy or indulgent.

Do any of these feel familiar? How do you feel about the idea of rest? This microgain will challenge your ideas on rest and ask you to see it as something that can benefit you, help your mood, make you more productive and efficient, and less stressed, exhausted and overwhelmed.

Rest can mean many things. Rest can be both active and non-active. It can be with others or alone. It can be a few minutes or a few hours. It can be anything that calms, soothes and restores you. Finding out what type of rest works for you and how you can incorporate this into your day is crucial. The most important thing is that it should feel restful and restorative.

TYPES OF REST

There are seven common types of rest which we can explore:[11]

1. **Physical** – Allowing your body to find rest or relaxation. For example: sleeping, laying down, doing gentle yoga stretches, having a massage, slow walking.
2. **Mental** – Allowing your mind to rest. For example: watching something easy on TV, taking breaks from work/admin tasks (anything requiring a lot of thinking), meditating, choosing strategies to set down worries or step away from negative thoughts/rumination, *giving yourself permission to stop/take a break.*
3. **Spiritual** – Allowing yourself to connect to something greater than you. This might be through religion, meditation, or other spiritual practices that bring meaning and purpose into your life.
4. **Emotional** – Allowing yourself to talk, write, express your emotions in healthy ways (e.g., journaling, therapy, talking to friends, family or loved ones); stepping away from situations that are causing you significant stress; enabling yourself to have rest/breaks from emotionally challenging situations or experiences.
5. **Social** – Allowing yourself a rest from social demands, or making choices to be in the company of people who make you feel relaxed and re-energized.
6. **Creative** – Allowing yourself to either have a break from being creative (if you are doing this all day) or allowing yourself to rest by engaging in a creative activity that soothes and restores you. This could be knitting, crocheting, painting, drawing, doodling, playing music, dancing or baking.
7. **Sensory** – Allowing your senses to rest. For example, turning off the radio/TV or only listening to very soothing music; turning lights down or off and lying in a dark or dimmed space; using calming scents like lavender.

MICROGAIN CHALLENGE

Choose (at least) one of the seven areas where you know you would benefit from rest.

Give yourself permission to find rest. Schedule when you can create this rest time and do this. Notice how it feels afterwards.

TOP TIP

Giving yourself full **permission** to rest is vital. Without this permission, we might look like we are resting, but with an inner voice full of "you should be working", "you should be doing something", it won't be restful.

MICROGAIN 4.3

IMPROVE YOUR SLEEP ROUTINE

Sleep is crucial for physical and mental health – and brain health. We know that sleep impacts mood, thinking skills, hormones, weight, energy levels and motivation. Yet despite most of us knowing all the benefits it brings, it's often something we don't get enough of, and one of the first things to suffer when things become stressful.

Creating conditions for good sleep is a small thing we can do to help us move toward better sleep. In this microgain, we'll consider two areas we can focus on:

1. Creating a sleep-conducive environment
2. Creating a wind-down routine to encourage our bodies and minds to be ready for sleep once we get into bed

CREATING A SLEEP-CONDUCIVE ENVIRONMENT

Here are some ideas to help you create a good environment for sleep (also called sleep hygiene):

- Use your bed/bedroom only for sleep, rest and sex. Try your best not to use it for work, study or anything that will make you associate it with being awake.
- Do what you can to make it dark enough, a suitable temperature for you (not too cold or too hot), and comfortable (weighted duvets, light sheets – whatever comfort means for you).

- Don't eat or drink too close to bed. This reduces the chance that you will need the bathroom in the night.
- Make your bed and tidy your room in the morning or earlier in the day, so that when you go to bed you are coming into a calming space.
- Reduce phone/screen use at bedtime. Consider a book or listen to an audiobook or sleep app.

CREATING A WIND-DOWN ROUTINE

Your wind-down routine will look different to someone else's. Consider the below, and choose at least three steps to create your routine.

- Go to bed when you begin to feel sleepy/at similar time each day.
- Turn off your phone/screen at least 20 minutes before sleep.
- Brush your teeth.
- Do a calming yoga stretch.
- Read a book.
- Listen to relaxing music.
- Do an evening meditation.
- Use a scented pillow spray or eye mask.

MICROGAIN CHALLENGE

Decide on one thing that will help create good conditions for your sleep and one thing you can do to slowly wind down toward sleep.
Commit to making these changes tonight.

TOP TIP

Take some time to look at your current sleep routine. Is there anything that works well? Is there anything you would consider to be unhelpful? Use this as a starting point to make changes to your sleep routine.

MICROGAIN 4.4

GET TO (OR BACK TO) SLEEP

Getting to sleep or getting back to sleep is a skill we can all develop. It is very common to wake intermittently throughout the night and fall back to sleep without even realizing this has happened. However, if you do struggle to sleep, fall asleep or get back to sleep on waking, this microgain is for you.

Exploring what is keeping you awake is important. You can then look to find a solution. Consider if any of the common reasons we might struggle to sleep/fall back to sleep apply to you:

1. Ruminating on worries or anxious thoughts
2. Thinking about aspects of the day, your life, situations (perhaps not categorized as worries, but preoccupying your mind nevertheless)
3. Worrying about not sleeping
4. Being uncomfortable (too hot/cold, feeling pain/unwell/aches)
5. Needing the toilet
6. The effect of hormones or blood sugars
7. Sleep cycles and rhythms
8. Being woken by children/pets
9. Sharing a bed with someone who wakes frequently or snores

TACKLING WHAT IS KEEPING US AWAKE

Thinking-related issues
For any thinking- or worry-related issues (points 1–3 above), follow these steps at the time you are struggling with sleep:

- As soon as you notice yourself worrying/thinking/pondering, see if you can stop, pause and ask yourself: "Do I need to spend time on this? If I do, can I write this down so I can deal with this in the morning?" Do this if needed, making a note on a notepad (or if there's no notepad available, note it on your phone, but please use screens as a last resort and try to look at them as briefly as possible).
- Be gentle but firm with yourself that thinking about this at this time of night will only make you feel worse and keep you awake. Aim to refocus (below) to help yourself get back to sleep as quickly as possible.
- Consider any of the following:
  - Trying a breathing exercise (Microgain 2.2)
  - Meditating, specifically with a sleep meditation (the Calm app has some great sleep stories and meditations)
  - Imagining being on a relaxing holiday – imagine in detail what you can see, hear, touch, taste and smell
  - Listening to calming music

Toilet visits

- Experiment with not drinking too close to bedtime. Chart the difference that bringing your last drink back by half an hour a night has on any waking.
- If you do have to get up for the toilet, try to do this (safely) with dim lights. Don't look at your phone, and try to settle back into bed as quickly as possible.

Comfort-related issues

Consider practical or medical (pain-management) solutions that will alleviate your symptoms, and manage your comfort-related issues as best you can. Please also seek advice from a medical practitioner.

Hormones

If you suspect your hormones may be playing a part in your issues sleeping – especially if you have been experiencing perimenopausal or menopausal symptoms – then do seek appropriate advice and support from your doctor or specialist practitioner.

MICROGAIN CHALLENGE

Prepare strategies to help your night's sleep.
Identify a breathing exercise, a sleep meditation, a book and/or a podcast that you can call upon easily the next time you need help getting to sleep, or after waking up in the middle of the night. Add a notepad to your bedside table for note-taking.

TOP TIP

If you wake in the night and have been lying awake in bed for more than about 20 minutes, then get out of bed and sit in a chair/sofa or a room nearby, and read a magazine or book with a low-level reading light for a while, or do some gentle breathing. Wait until you feel sleepy to go back to bed. Do not lie in bed awake for long periods, becoming stressed about not sleeping, as this can create an unhelpful association between your bed and not sleeping.

MICROGAIN 4.5

REDUCE ALCOHOL AND CAFFEINE

Two big disruptors of sleep and rest are alcohol and caffeine. Studies have shown that alcohol is linked to poor-quality sleep and a decrease in sleep duration. Alcohol impacts sleep in this way even when a person consumes only few drinks, with the problematic effects increasing with the amount of alcohol consumed.[12] Caffeine promotes wakefulness and disrupts sleepiness. It blocks the production of adenosine, which is a chemical that encourages sleep.[13] Caffeine and alcohol use can also interfere with rest during the day, as they can make us feel jittery, anxious and unsettled.

HOW MUCH IS YOUR INTAKE?

- It's recommended that you have up to 400mg of caffeine a day. That's approximately four small cups of coffee or eight cups of tea. For good sleep, ideally consume your caffeine before lunchtime/mid-afternoon.
- It's recommended that you have up to 14 units of alcohol per week (one unit = approximately one small glass of wine or half a pint of low-strength beer). Even one or two units per day has been found to impact sleep quality.

Add up approximately how many caffeinated drinks you are taking in each day and over a week. How often do you drink these from lunchtime onward?

Add up approximately how much alcohol you are taking in each day and over a week, too.

Be as honest as you can – you don't have to share this with anyone; it's for your wellbeing alone.

Given your answers to the above, are there any changes you would like to make? What would you like to commit to and why?

There are, of course, wider reasons that you might consider reducing your alcohol and caffeine intake beyond sleep and rest alone. These might include addiction issues, social consequences, physical health, cognitive functioning, weight and mood. If you think there are wider reasons to address these issues, please do seek help and support.

IDEAS FOR REDUCING CAFFEINE

- Alternate caffeinated and decaffeinated coffee when making or buying drinks.
- Reduce your consumption from two shots to one shot of espresso.
- Limit caffeine after lunchtime. Not consuming after 4pm is recommended for good sleep.
- Have days without caffeine or choose decaffeinated options.

IDEAS FOR REDUCING ALCOHOL

- Set a reduced plan and/or budget for your alcohol use – at home and when socializing.
- Dilute your alcoholic drink with things like soda water or non-alcoholic drinks, or drink water in between alcoholic drinks.
- Choose to add an alcohol-free day into your schedule. If you already have some of these days, what happens if you add another?
- Consider why you drink. Does this connect with the person you want to be? Do you drink for the taste or because of how

it makes you feel? Alcohol is a disinhibitor and can give us the illusion of feeling more relaxed in social situations. We can also overly rely on it to help us feel less anxious, even though it has been found to cause increased levels of anxiety.

- Reducing alcohol use at home or in certain situations can be easier to begin with. Consider where the easiest place to start would be.

MICROGAIN CHALLENGE

Choose one small way to reduce your caffeine or alcohol intake today.

Make it small, specific and possible to begin now.

TOP TIP

Start by focusing on one area at a time, for example, your alcohol consumption. Be kind to yourself as you reduce your intake, as behavioural changes take time to implement.

CHAPTER 5

SOCIAL CONNECTION MICROGAINS

"Connection is why we're here... it's what gives purpose and meaning to our lives."

"Connection is the energy that exists between people when they feel seen, heard and valued."[14]

Brené Brown, writer and professor

THE MICROGAINS

1. Make a Connection or Reconnection
2. Forge a Human–Animal Connection
3. Draw a Connection Tree
4. Enhance or Re-evaluate Connections
5. Put Your Phone Down

Social psychology – the study of human behaviour – has shown that humans are social creatures who are driven to connect, to belong in groups, to exist within a community. The role of connection in our ability to thrive and survive is central to who we are.

An important report by the New Economics Foundation on the Five Ways to Wellbeing also highlights the importance of connection:

"Connect: With the people around you. With family, friends, colleagues and neighbours. At home, work, school or in your local community. Think of these as the cornerstones of your life and invest time in developing them. Building these connections will support and enrich you every day."[15]

Connection may mean many things. Connections may be about:

• The people you connect with – family, friends, colleagues or people you meet in your community
• The connections you have with pets, groups, communities or through hobbies
• Different types of connection – social connections, religious or spiritual connections, physical connections, lighter moments or intimate, deeper ones
• The connection you have with yourself – understanding yourself, being compassionate to yourself and the awareness you have within yourself

Connection can have many benefits including lifting your mood, improving self-esteem and physical health, reducing loneliness, increasing empathy and enhancing cooperation with others.

Whether you see yourself as an introvert or an extrovert, connection is still meaningful, although it is, of course, individual for each of us as to what exactly this looks like. Some may thrive from being part of large groups, others may enjoy one-to-one connections; some may enjoy constant social interaction, whereas others may prefer a slower pace of connection.

MICROGAIN 5.1

MAKE A CONNECTION OR RECONNECTION

In this fast-paced, ever-changing world, it is easy to become a little disconnected from those around you. Days and weeks can go by before you realize that you haven't checked in with a friend or phoned a parent, or that you haven't seen someone important to you for a long time.

A lovely way to connect to yourself and others is to take action to make some purposeful connection. This connection can make you feel less alone and instead part of a group or community. It can increase feelings of belonging, love, care and humour, and provide a sense of achievement or satisfaction for checking in.

HOW TO CONNECT

Ask yourself:

- Who are your valued connections?
- Who are the people who make you feel good about yourself?
- Who do you have shared values with?
- Who do you want to continue to have in your life?
- Is there someone you haven't connected with in a while?
- Have you been putting off – or have you just not gotten round to – messaging, replying to or meeting up with someone?

- What could be the value in reconnecting with them?
- What are the barriers in reaching out? How can these be overcome?

Then begin to ask yourself:

- Can you make a connection plan?
- Who will you start with?
- What will the communication method be?
  - Send a text
  - Send a little card
  - Make a phone call
  - Reach out on social media
- What will you say?

MICROGAIN CHALLENGE

Choose one person to reconnect with and consider the best way you can do this.
This might be someone who is regularly in your life, but you've been slow responding to their messages with this week, or it might be someone you've lost connection with some time ago. Whoever you choose, take action and make that connection today.

TOP TIP

It can sometimes feel daunting to reconnect with someone again. If you find the thought of a meet-up or telephone call difficult, then consider reaching out by message or social media with a like or a comment on a photo. You can then build up to more intensive contact when you are ready.

MICROGAIN 5.2

FORGE A HUMAN–ANIMAL CONNECTION

Spending time with animals has been proven to bring mental and physical health benefits. This can include improved mood, lower anxiety and stress, lower cortisol levels, increased serotonin and dopamine (feel-good chemicals), reduced blood pressure and improved cardiovascular functioning. It has also been shown to lead to a reduction in loneliness and an increase in exercise and playfulness. These benefits have been found through:

- Owning a loved pet
- Stroking/petting animals/pets
- Spending time with animals in the community

OWNING A PET

Owning a pet can bring a sense of companionship, connection and support. It has been determined that dogs, for example, can try and read your emotional state and offer comfort.[16] Owning a pet can provide opportunities for physical activity, exercise and play. It can also create a reason to go outside and be in nature and the fresh air. Studies have also shown that owning a pet can lead to less trips to the doctor for those over the age of 65.[17]

If you have the privilege of being able to find the time, space and finances to afford a pet, explore how you can bring the benefits of being a pet owner into your daily life. This might mean carving out specific time for your pet, amongst the business of normal life.

ACCESS TO ANIMALS

Not all of us are in the position to be able to afford a pet, or practically look after or manage a pet, no matter how much we might like one or see the benefits. So what can we do instead? Here are some ideas:

- Spend time with friends' or family pets
- Offer to look after or walk friends'/family/neighbours' dogs
- Try a puppy yoga class
- Visit an animal shelter/farm/petting zoo
- Volunteer at an animal shelter
- Offer to take care of pets when their owners are away (or perhaps become a professional pet sitter!)
- Try a scheme such as BorrowMyDoggy
- Have a horse-riding lesson
- Find a dog or cat café
- Consider fostering a pet

MICROGAIN CHALLENGE

Pick one of the ideas above or come up with your own small way to create a human–animal connection.

Whichever route you choose to enhance your human–animal connection, spend time with your chosen animal slowly, gently and mindfully. Take your time in the moment to be present. Allow yourself to just be.

TOP TIP

Animals can create powerful connections with humans and can teach us so much. When connecting with animals, observe their energy. As you get to know them more, you will get to know their moods and further enhance your connection.

MICROGAIN 5.3

DRAW A CONNECTION TREE

Feeling connected with others helps increase our sense of belonging. Due to the nature of the social network-based world we live in, we may all have more connections that we realize. Try this microgain to explore and enhance your awareness of this.

DRAW YOUR CONNECTION TREE

- Take a moment to consider the connections in your life.
- Now grab a pen and paper and sketch out the trunk of a tree with branches. (It doesn't have to be exact or pretty – no judgement on your art skills!)
- Begin to add the names of the connections in your life on the branches of the tree – these can range from people you know as very casual acquaintances (e.g., school friends from Facebook), to casual day-to-day acquaintances, to closer friends and intimate relationships. This may include all or any of the following people: neighbours, community contacts, colleagues, friends (old and new), family members, relatives, partners.
- If you are getting stuck with this exercise, it can help to look at your phone contacts or your social media pages to remind yourself of the connections in your life.

This exercise can help you identify the range of connections in your life. It may help you identify:

- Connections you have forgotten

- Connections you haven't been in touch with for a while and with whom you would like to reconnect
- Which connections are most meaningful or important for you
- Areas in which you would like to expand or increase your connections by creating new ones

However this works for you is okay.

After reflecting on what your connection tree means for you, see if you can identify one action you can take that will 1) add, or 2) increase, or 3) build a connection, or 4) create a new branch in some way. Building new connections or new branches may look like, for example, joining a club or group with shared interests of yours, or considering online dating or friendship apps to create new connections. It may also mean initiating increased connection with people you already know.

MICROGAIN CHALLENGE

Draw out your connection tree and choose someone to connect with today.

Use the tree to continue maintaining connections with people you already have on the tree, or focus on new connections you want to make to add to the tree.

TOP TIP

When you are feeling lonely or stuck for how to engage or make a connection socially, have a look at your connection tree for inspiration as to who to get in contact with, or for ideas to build connection.

MICROGAIN 5.4

ENHANCE OR RE-EVALUATE CONNECTIONS

Social connections can bring us joy, support, love and a sense of belonging. Enhancing and encouraging these connections in our lives wholly benefits us. At the same time, social connections can also negatively impact our mental health at times. This might happen when a friendship/relationship:

- Is one-sided in what it offers, or the support it brings
- Causes you more stress or unhappiness than it brings you joy
- Suffers from unhealthy boundaries
- Contains any elements of unkindness, bullying or, ultimately, abuse

Making steps to re-evaluate and create healthy boundaries in relationships that do not serve you can be very important for your wellbeing.

It is okay to revise a relationship. It can be a positive thing to change or end a relationship. It is okay to let go and still hold fond memories. Friendships and relationships can sometimes run their course, be time-limited, or have an important place at certain times in our lives and play less of a role in others. Relationships and friendships can also be, or become, unhealthy or harmful.

We are always growing and changing; sometimes our relationships grow with us, and sometimes they don't. Just because something worked once doesn't mean it will be working now.

Whatever the situation, we know that we can often stay in relationships longer than they benefit us – perhaps because of thinking about what we "should" do or what others expect of us, or due to not wanting to cause upset or conflict, or not quite knowing how to go about change.

HOW TO EVALUATE A RELATIONSHIP

Start by thinking about the people in your life (reflect on your connection tree, Microgain 5.3). Do a check-in for each relationship. This can feel awkward at first – let yourself reflect on one at a time and ask yourself:

- What do I like?
- What don't I like?
- How do I feel in this relationship?
- Do I like myself and the other person in this relationship?
- Would I like to enhance this relationship or re-evaluate/ revise it?
- (Difficult question) Does this relationship work still?
- Are there reasons that the relationship is struggling right now that are to do with me and/or the other person's wants/needs/ values?
- Are there outside stressors (divorce, physical or mental health issues, loss, financial/work worries) that are affecting the relationship?
- Have our support needs for each other changed in this relationship?
- Am I happy with the shared boundaries in this relationship?
- How could things be different?
- What is the most healthy and compassionate way to understand and re-evaluate this relationship?

SMALL STEPS TO TAKE TO ENHANCE OR REVISE A CONNECTION

If a relationship is to be revised, what does this look like? Consider your options: ending the relationship, working on improving the relationship or changing the relationship into a different form (for example, into a less-intense friendship). Whatever you do, lead with kindness and compassion.

Next steps might include:

- Resolving to message/communicate differently – more or less frequently, and/or with a different method (for example, by email or WhatsApp, or with more phone calls)
- Organizing a coffee/walk/drink to improve time together or talk about an aspect of the relationship
- Making a decision to do one thing differently in the relationship
- Seeking support from a charity or therapist, or exploring resources on relationships to help you understand yourself and the situation
- Learning more about assertiveness or healthy boundaries and what these can look like

MICROGAIN CHALLENGE

Take time to reflect on a friendship, relationship or connection in your life.

Ask yourself the questions in this microgain and consider: what small step could you take today to enhance or revise this relationship in a compassionate and healthy way?

TOP TIP

Be compassionate toward yourself when reflecting on the relationships in your life. Feelings such as guilt and negative self-judgement can lead us to feel that we shouldn't revise or end relationships that don't work for us. Remember, it can take time to work through your feelings, but the more you are able to set boundaries and revise your relationships, the easier this will become.

MICROGAIN 5.5

PUT YOUR PHONE DOWN

Modern technology is presenting us with more and more challenges every day. For ourselves, for our children, for our relationships. The fast pace, the notifications, the constant availability. It is becoming harder to focus, to engage in one activity – on a TV show or movie, on one conversation – without a glance at a phone, a new message, notification, email; without the temptation to show something you have seen when scrolling.

Our phone use can frequently get in the way of our relationships with others. It can interrupt our attention and focus on conversations, it can pause interactions when we are distracted by our phones, and it can make people feel unheard or unimportant. Relationships between couples, friends, and children and their parents can often become disconnected in both directions when phone use gets in the way.

Taking time away from our devices can also benefit our mental and physical health. We know this includes better sleep, focus and productivity, reduced stress and boosted mood, alongside improved relationships with others.

Take a moment to reflect on how often phone use interferes with your relationships. Do you notice interactions being paused, interrupted or disconnected due to your phone use or others' phone use? Do you notice yourself tuning out of interactions as you look at your phone instead – intentionally or not? Do you find yourself able to keep your phone out of sight when you are socializing?

CHANGING YOUR PHONE USE

Putting your phone down and increasing connection could look like:

- Putting your phone out of reach/sight during social occasions
- Agreeing and modelling no screen/phone at mealtimes and putting your phone out of sight
- Having a weekend/morning/evening/day with loved ones with no screens/phones
- Turning your phone on silent or turning off notifications when you want to focus on your interactions
- Letting key people know you will not be available during specific hours due to social commitments, and being off your phone at these times

When you do this, see if you can notice:

- How it feels to have this screen-/phone-free time
- How you engage with relationships and activities in this time
- How it affects your ability to feel connected
- How it affects your ability to feel present
- How it affects your ability to engage in the world around you

MICROGAIN CHALLENGE

Choose one way that you can create a screen-/phone-free time with the goal of improving your connections and interactions each day.

Choose the easiest place you can implement this at first. You can continue to expand this over time if/as you like. Choose one specific way to do this today.

TOP TIP

Observe your phone behaviour for a few days. Do you notice how it interferes with your relationships? Do you notice a particular time of day when your use increases or is more problematic in some way? For example, you may realize you scroll more when commuting to work or when going to bed. Focus on this as an area of change.

CHAPTER 6

MOVEMENT MICROGAINS

"The most important thing is to remain active and to love what you are doing."[18]

Leslie Caron, actress and dancer

THE MICROGAINS

1. Sit, Stand, Stretch
2. Explore the Movement of Yoga
3. Just Walk
4. Set Yourself an Active Challenge
5. Change Your Posture

Moving your body, as most of us know, is great for your emotional and physical health. What you might *not* know is that it is also good for enhancing your cognitive abilities, self-confidence and self-esteem. And being active regularly can improve mood, reduce anxiety and stress, reduce high blood pressure, improve sleep, improve decision making and much more.

Before we go any further, let's acknowledge that for some of us, the idea of movement, exercise and being active can feel like something we immediately resist. You might have grown up being made to do compulsory exercise, or bullied or criticized into working out when it was last thing you wanted to do. You may have come to associate everything movement-based or active as negative. If this is you, please bear with us.

Firstly, the microgains included are small, manageable and chosen to help you explore what works for you. Secondly, we believe movement should be enjoyable. This is about enhancing your mental health and wellbeing in positive ways.

Movement and being active can mean many things, and we hope to inspire you with some ideas. Movement microgains may take the shape of:

- **Formal or typical exercise routes** – such as strenuous/ intense exercise, sport, weights or cardio-based activities
- **Activity-based exercise** – such as dancing, trampolining, gymnastics, ballet, acrobatics or surfing
- **Less intense/low-impact or gentler activities** – such as walking, stretching, swimming or yoga
- **Everyday activities** – such as shopping, doing chores, visiting historical sites of interest, picking up your kids at school or gardening

It is important to highlight that moving your body and being active can look very different for different people, and what each person finds enjoyable will vary too.

The key message here is that this section is about finding a way of being active and moving your body that *you* find enjoyable – or could learn to love – that inspires you, motivates you and energizes you. This is important to stress as it's common for people to believe that there can only be gains from doing formal or intense exercise, and they may have never been supported enough to enjoy being active in a positive way.

We are also very mindful this section may be orientated in parts to able-bodied people. We hope that the ideas in each section can be adapted, or may prompt inspiration, for you to introduce more movement into your life, in ways that work for you.

Please note: This section is not intended to replace professional guidance in respect to being medically able to partake in physical movement. If you are in doubt, please consult your physical health practitioner.

MICROGAIN 6.1

SIT, STRETCH, STAND

How much time do you spend being stationary or sitting at your desk? How much time do you spend feeling stiff, achy, or less mobile or flexible than you might like? Being able to find opportunities to move your body in gentle ways, to create breaks from sitting, to create more movement, flexibility, and to reduce tension and stiffness are all small things that will make a difference to the way your body and mind feel.

Please seek the advice of a medical or physical health practitioner if needed before engaging in any exercise or movement plan.

SIMPLE MOVEMENT

If you have been in one position too long, take some simple action to move your body into different positions. This might be simply sitting or standing in a different position. It might be a gentle movement around the room – from sitting to standing, to doing a stretch or even having a little dance.

SIMPLE CHAIR-BASED STRETCHES

These are simple exercises you can do in your chair, at home, at your desk or at your computer.

Arm raises

- Sit in a chair with your feet shoulder-width apart. Take your shoes off if you can. Feel the ground beneath your feet.

- Sit upright and look straight ahead.
- Position your chair so you are looking at an image that you like.
- Slowly raise your arms above your head and stretch out your fingers. Give your fingers a wiggle if you like.
- Hold for a few seconds before lowering.
- Repeat five times.

Gentle bends

- Raise your arms above your head as in the exercise above, but this time gently bend your arms and body to the right slowly.
- Come back upright and then bend slowly to the left.
- Repeat five times.

Head turns

- Sit in a chair, with your arms by your side. Gently continue to sit upright.
- Slowly turn your head to the right and notice what you can see.
- Come back to the centre, then slowly turn your head to the left and notice what you can see.
- Repeat five times.

Sit to stand

- Sit in a chair, with both feet on the floor. Try to stand without using your hands if possible.
- Move slowly to standing and then sit down again.
- Repeat five times.

Forward leans

- Sit in a chair and place your hands on your legs.
- Slowly lean forward as far as you can with a straight back and then return to sitting upright.
- Repeat five times.

STANDING MOVEMENT

- If you are spending a lot of time sitting down, slowly stand up.
- Start with gently creating a little movement in your body – rotate your shoulders, give your arms and legs a little gentle shake. Take a big, deep breath.
- With your arms by your side, gently move them out to the sides in a sweeping circle until they come together above your head. Hold for a moment then gently move them down again. Breathe in as you lift your arms up, breathe out as you lower your arms down.
- Repeat three times.

MICROGAIN CHALLENGE

Notice how your body is doing and how often you have moved in the last hour.
Choose one of these small movements or stretches to try today.

TOP TIP

Choose a stretch that fits your needs. Are you noticing any aches or stiffness in your body from sitting? Do you need to sit or stand? Where do you need to focus right now? Choose an exercise that targets that area.

MICROGAIN 6.2

EXPLORE THE MOVEMENT OF YOGA

The practice of yoga has been found to be beneficial for our mental health, physical health and wellbeing. The words "yoga asana" are used to describe the practices or poses of yoga. Many of us know yoga can be good for us, and many of us love to incorporate this into our days. If you already do, that's wonderful! Feel free to adapt this microgain however you feel is helpful from your experience. If you haven't yet found a way to incorporate yoga into your world, this microgain shows you one small way you can incorporate a yoga pose into a few minutes of your day, with positive effect.

Please note: This yoga pose has been recommended by a qualified and experienced yoga teacher, Diane Shepherd, but it is always advisable to check with a doctor or suitably trained physical health professional if you are in any doubt that yoga, or any pose, would be suitable for you to do.

LEGS-UP-THE-WALL POSE

You've probably heard the expression, "Take the load off" – this simple yoga pose is a way to do just that. Legs-Up-the-Wall, or *Viparita Karani* in Sanskrit, is a restorative pose used to let go of stress, anxiety and tension, and to restore energy and calm into your body. It has been reported to improve circulation and calm tension headaches. It can be a wonderful pose as part of your bedtime wind-down routine.

The key to this pose is to feel comfortable enough so you can melt into the floor.

- Find a quiet and warm space near a bare wall where you can lie on your back on a comfortable surface. You may experiment with cushions or rolled-up towels under your back or head to find what works for you. You may want to relax your arms by your side or have them outstretched.
- Sit facing the wall. Then slowly lower your back and head to the floor.
- Gently move yourself into a position where your legs are vertical up against the wall, your bottom is resting close to the point where the wall meets the floor, and your back is lying in a horizontal line along the floor. This should look like you are forming an L with your body.
- The aim is to be able to rest in the pose for up to 20 minutes, but just start with a few minutes today. The aim is for the wall to support your legs, and you should not need to make any effort to hold them against the wall.
- You might move around a little bit to find your position. When you have found that comfortable position, then you can begin to focus on your breath and relax your mind.
- If at any time you experience discomfort, it is important to adjust your position.
- Come out of this position by slowly bending your knees and turning over onto your side.
- Always come out of a yoga posture slowly and safely.

MICROGAIN CHALLENGE

Could you try this right now? Or could you plan it into your diary to try when you get home, before bed or any other time?
If you like this pose, can you plan to incorporate it into your regular routine? Or consider trying another yoga pose or adapt one to suit your physical abilities? If you are experienced at yoga, is there another pose you would like to incorporate into your day/week?

TOP TIP

Take your time with any yoga pose you try. Move gently and slowly, and breathe deeply. With each breath, see if you can ease into the pose or the stretch a little more.

MICROGAIN 6.3

JUST WALK

Walking might just be one of the most underrated ways for an able-bodied person to move their body and be active. It is something you can do for free, that you can do anywhere and immediately, without any special equipment, and that helps improve physical and mental health. For most able-bodied people without injuries, this is the simplest low-intensity movement-based activity.

Not only is walking fairly easy for us to do, it is also incredibly beneficial. Walking can improve physical health, brain function, productivity, resilience, mental health and emotional wellbeing. It can also prevent cognitive decline. Regular short walks of 15 minutes can improve concentration and memory, decrease levels of stress and anxiety, and improve mood and resilience. The rhythmic movement created when walking can lead to more effective emotional processing and decision making.

You can reap even more benefits by taking your walks in green spaces. Walking in nature can lower blood pressure and heart rate, decrease levels of stress, and improve mood and general cognition.

WALK MORE

There are lots of different ways to incorporate walking into your life. Today, try taking a longer route to school/work/the park. Or, instead of meeting a friend for a coffee, plan a walk instead.

There are also many ways to make walking into a more formal activity, which appeals to some people. This could include counting steps, aiming to increase your mileage per week, or taking on a walking challenge for charity or personal achievement.

Even a ten-minute walk can improve your mood. Get some comfy shoes on, plug yourself into a podcast and go round the block. See how you feel afterwards. We bet you won't regret it.

MICROGAIN CHALLENGE

How can you incorporate walking a little more (or a lot more) into: a) right now? b) some point today? c) your week?
Make a commitment to one small way you can do this. If you can act right now, do it! If you can plan it today, schedule this into your diary or phone. If you can plan it this week, do the same – and stick to it!

TOP TIP

Consider any small way you can increase your walking/steps in your day. This could be at home, whilst communing or shopping, or with friends. Take small steps to choose walking where you can.

MICROGAIN 6.4

SET YOURSELF AN ACTIVE CHALLENGE

Setting ourselves a challenge can inspire and motivate us, and lift our moods. Setting a (reasonable) active challenge gives us a focus and the opportunity to gain a sense of achievement, as well as all the benefits that the activity/movement/exercise brings itself.

An active challenge could be an organized event, or something you set yourself. It might include:

- Deciding to walk up the stairs instead of using the lift or escalator
- Skipping rope for five minutes a day
- Walking to and from the station instead of taking a cab/bus
- Committing to standing up and walking around your office/home/garden/school at least once an hour, especially when you're very stationary in your day
- Cycling to work
- Walking, jogging or cycling X miles per day/week/month/year
- Dancing to a song on the radio each morning
- Doing a set of star jumps or press-ups every time you wait for kettle to boil
- Adding a 30-second sprint to your regular jog
- Signing up for an active charity challenge (a walk, cycle, marathon, triathlon, hike, swim-a-thon...)
- Doing a yoga pose, flow or Pilates routine every morning
- Embarking on a DIY project that involves being active
- Learning a new active hobby (dancing, sailing, horse riding, paddleboarding, kayaking...)

- Training for a challenge – to climb a significant hill or mountain, to walk a coastal path or river length, to jog the equivalent distance of one end of the country to the other...

TIPS FOR AN ACTIVE CHALLENGE

- Make it specific. What exactly are you going to do?
- Set a timescale – one week, one month, six months, etc.
- Schedule it in your diary. When are you going to do this challenge? What time of day, which days of the week?
- Identify your reason or motivation for the challenge and write this down. For example: to be more active, to move more, to improve your physical health and/or mental health, to lift your energy levels or mood, to gain a sense of achievement, to raise money for charity, to give you a focus, etc.
- Identify any barriers to this challenge and problem-solve these.
- Make it public. Let people know about your challenge, and make your commitment public.
- Don't give up. Life inevitably gets in the way at times; look at how to get back on track and do this as soon as you can.

MICROGAIN CHALLENGE

Choose an active challenge that works for you.
Set yourself a specific challenge using the steps above.

TOP TIP

Remember, in accordance with the microgain concept, this can be a *really small challenge for just five minutes in your day.*

MICROGAIN 6.5

CHANGE YOUR POSTURE

A simple tool we can use to create a shift in how we feel is to make a change to our body posture or stance. When we change how our bodies are positioned, we can create lifts in mood, beyond what we might expect. Once we discover the impact of making small shifts in facial expression, posture or pose, it is possible to use this when we need a boost – for example, before walking into a meeting, while walking down the street or getting out of bed. Try any of the below.

FACIAL AND POSTURE CHANGES

Let's start with changing your facial expression. With a very straight, serious face say to yourself, "Hi, how are you?" Now with a big smile and lots of energy, repeat, "Hi, how are you?" How do you feel? What differences in your energy level and in your body do you notice?

Now let's try your posture. Whatever you are doing right now, start by slumping your shoulders, looking at the ground, maybe crossing your arms. Now take a breath and see if you can straighten your back, look straight ahead, hold your shoulders back, and uncross your arms or legs. Smooth out your face, un-wrinkle your brow. Let a slight smile appear on your lips. Look around you with this open posture. Breathe. How does this feel?

Now let's make it bigger. From a standing or seated position, lift your arms up above your head as if you have just won a race or been awarded a gold medal and are standing on the podium. Imagine lifting your arms up and saying "YES!" as you cheer for yourself with a little smile. Notice what happens in your body and your mood/energy.

Now try moving into a warrior pose: strong stance, hands on hips, chin lifted up, shoulders back. Take a deep breath. How does this feel?

MICROGAIN CHALLENGE

Find a quiet spot and try the above movements today.

Identify one place in your day/week where you could incorporate this microgain.

TOP TIP

Try this right now – change your facial expression to neutral, angry, happy. Then say, "Hi, how are you?" in each of the different expressions. Notice the difference in how it feels.

CHAPTER 7

PURPOSEFUL ACTION MICROGAINS

"When you do the things in the present that you can see, you are shaping the future that you are yet to see."[19]

Idowu Koyenikan, change consultant

THE MICROGAINS

1. Do Something Silly/Adventurous/Pleasurable
2. Do Something You've Been Putting Off
3. Get Help with a Problem
4. Plan Ahead
5. Dance Like No One's Watching!

There are times in life when we need to slow down, and there are times when we need to take action. When an action has the possibility of moving us in a different, positive direction, we need to take notice. Sometimes this is just a small step toward something important for us; sometimes it is tackling a task we have been putting off.

At times of overwhelm or stress, we can become stuck in inaction. Avoidance and procrastination can dominate, and our mental health can suffer because of it. Finding ways to tackle inaction can be a very helpful skill to develop.

Equally important is finding time for planning and engaging in enjoyable, mood-boosting activities – this is also something that can easily become side-lined.

So, in this section you'll find small ways to incorporate committed action into your life – to help make plans, add fun and pleasure, book things to look forward to, and also tackle those essential tasks you keep postponing or avoiding.

MICROGAIN 7.1

DO SOMETHING SILLY/ ADVENTUROUS/PLEASURABLE

It's very easy to become caught up in everyday demands and activities. This is your call to take some time out of your normal routine, perhaps to step outside of your comfort zone and engage in some activities that are a bit different.

These can be activities that make you feel energized, alive, adventurous, like you're fully living life. What this looks like could be different for everyone. Often tuning into your values helps (see Microgain 10.2) – is it important to live with fun in your life, with playfulness, silliness or adventure?

Please note: Sometimes we become so caught up in the seriousness and responsibility of adulthood, or growing up, that we forget to allow ourselves to have fun. In this microgain we really want you to challenge this.

IDEAS TO INSPIRE

Reading the ideas below, what inspires you?

- Doing something fun/silly/adventurous/exciting
- Doing something to challenge yourself, stepping out of your comfort zone
- Doing something that is outdoors or helps you meet new people
- Doing something completely different from your usual day to day

This might look impromptu, like:

- Playing children's games like hide-and-seek, mini Olympics or races (you don't need children to join in!)
- Having an impromptu kitchen disco
- Camping in the garden or front room
- Having a water/pillow fight
- Exploring a new area of where you live
- Going geocaching
- Creating an obstacle course in the garden/your home
- Making a fort or den in the front room
- Watching something funny on TV
- Listening to a comedy podcast

And with a bit more planning:

- Organizing a game of rounders/football/a scavenger hunt
- Roller-skating like you did when you were a kid!
- Trying an acrobatic class or go to a BMX track
- Going racing! Inflatable races/colour-run races/obstacle-course races
- Booking a water-park inflatable or ziplining activity
- Going to a comedy or music show
- Learning to dance/ride a horse/cycle/kayak/paddleboard/swim
- Skimming stones on the beach/by a river
- Exploring your local woods and making nature art with things you find

MICROGAIN CHALLENGE

Pick one idea from the list or come up with your own.

Write down why this idea appeals to you. Consider how it would feel to engage in this activity. Can you do this activity today? This week? Or can you begin to work through the steps to making plans?

TOP TIP

Imagine you are truly free to be you. Let your inner child out. Be silly, fun, playful, go on adventures. What can you do today to tap into this feeling?

MICROGAIN 7.2

DO SOMETHING YOU'VE BEEN PUTTING OFF

Our wellbeing can be negatively impacted when we become stationary, caught in procrastination and overwhelm. As these feelings intensify, we may begin putting off tasks. We may see a long to-do list at work, or come home to piles of chores, and end up feeling so overwhelmed, stuck or stressed that we can't quite face any of it. These feelings of stuckness and avoidance can easily build, and suddenly we are paralysed by the many tasks in front of us. This can quickly begin to negatively impact our mental health.

Can you identify any situations like this in your life? Are there things you are putting off? Tasks that have built up? To-dos that have been there for longer than you would like? People you have been meaning to message, reply to, call? Appointments you need to make or emails you need to sort through? Are there patterns where you get stuck and become less productive, and you notice this impacts your mood?

If this is you, ask yourself:

- Is there one task that you could action **right now** that you have been putting off?
- Is there one task that you have been putting off that you could schedule into your diary **right now** and commit to completing today or this week?
- If there is one task that you would love to tackle but you feel stuck, can you spend five minutes **right now** problem-solving a way forward?

- Is there a task you need to tackle that you need help or support with, and you could message/call/email someone **right now** to help with it?
- When you are sitting down, feeling stuck, procrastinating, what is the one thing you can say to yourself (**and make a note of right now**) to help yourself just get up and do the task? (Please note: This must be compassionately motivating, not critical, and it must also take into account when rest is absolutely appropriate.)
- Can you identify **at least one positive outcome** from which you will benefit if you complete this task/activity/chore/message?

TIPS TO DEAL WITH PROCRASTINATION AND PUTTING THINGS OFF

1. Don't wait until you *feel* like completing the task – just do it.
2. Make the task as specific as possible – what needs to be done, when, why, how, and with what support?
3. Remember: A task's completion might bring positive feelings of achievement, which will then help you with the next task.

MICROGAIN CHALLENGE

Choose one task/to-do list item today.

Take a step (or more) toward resolving it, following the ideas outlined above.

TOP TIP

In true alignment with the concept of microgains, START SMALL. Choose a task you think you can most easily tick off the list, or choose a small aspect of a task to start with. Build up from there.

MICROGAIN 7.3

GET HELP WITH A PROBLEM

At certain times in our lives, we may be juggling multiple issues or problems every day. At any one time, we might be dealing with issues related to any one (or more) of the following:

- Finances
- Work
- Physical health
- Mental health
- Relationships
- Parenting
- Schooling/studying
- Caring roles

When we are dealing with unresolved stressors and problems, this can, of course, negatively impact our mental health. However, we know it can be easy to delay dealing with a problem, and especially putting off asking for help. This may be because we lack time. It may be because we worry about or fear what will happen if we raise or tackle the problem. It may be because we've convinced ourselves we can manage it alone. It may stem from a fear of conflict. Whatever the reason, if you have an issue that you could resolve with some help, this microgain is for you.

SMALL STEPS TO TACKLE A PROBLEM

Consider any of the below:

1. Identify and acknowledge the problem.
2. Problem-solve. What is the problem? What solution are you aiming for? How do you think you can get there?
3. Acknowledge what might be stopping you from tackling the problem and consider what support you need to move forward.
4. Write down the benefits you will gain from solving the problem.
5. Consider what help and support you might need. This could be:
   - Self-help – books/articles/podcasts
   - Support from family/friends
   - Work-based help – colleagues/human resources/ occupational health
   - Help from a business professional – legal/administrative/ citizens advice/financial/business
   - Help from a tradesperson – DIY/home maintenance/car maintenance
   - Therapy-based help – medical/physical therapy/ psychological therapy/coaching
6. Research how you'd access this support. Find appropriate contact numbers/emails.
7. Break down the steps required to tackle the issue into small, manageable actions.
8. Make a specific plan to work through each step – What? When? Who? Where?
9. Take action, step by step.

MICROGAIN CHALLENGE

Identify a problem you want to address.

Read through the steps in this microgain and take at least one step today to begin to address the problem.

TOP TIP

If you get really stuck, slow down. Pause and problem-solve what you might need in order to move forward. If needed, take a break, and make a note in your diary of when you will next address this. Come back to this at your set time.

MICROGAIN 7.4

PLAN AHEAD

HAVE SOMETHING TO LOOK FORWARD TO

Being able to find contentment and happiness in the present moment is always important when it comes to our mental health. It's equally important to look to the future with hope and optimism. One small way we can do this is to plan things to look forward to.

Planning ahead and scheduling events into the diary can be a mood-boost in itself, and can also help combat procrastination or a lack of motivation. A solid plan makes something more likely to happen and reduces feelings of being solitary, stationary or stuck without plans.

What you might like to plan, and how far in advance you might like to plan, is completely up to you. You might like to plan:

- Something for this weekend, in a month's time or six months' time
- Something that involves being active – an adventure, challenge or new skill
- Something social that brings you more connection with others
- Something that enhances your relationships with people who are important to you
- Something that connects you with a hobby, passion or interest
- Something that brings you into nature
- Something that brings new environments or new experiences
- Something that helps you find joy, excitement, happiness or surprise

- Something that will make you feel relaxed, rested, restored and soothed
- Something that connects with an aspect of your faith, sexuality, culture or identity

IDEAS OF ACTIVITIES TO PLAN

- A weekend/week (or more) away – spa, travel, adventure, sea and sunshine
- Tourism – museum, stately home, cultural experience
- Theatre, musicals, plays, music and comedy gigs
- A retreat – health and wellness, faith-based
- Festivals or parades – music, literature, culture, faith, sexuality, identity, wellness
- Something fun/challenging/out of your comfort zone – escape room, high-wires, water parks, speedboat tours
- Children's entertainment – zoos, farms, adventure parks
- Academic or hobby-centric courses – learn something new

MICROGAIN CHALLENGE

Identify one activity to plan or make a list of your top three activities to plan over the next year.

Consider what it would be like if you could include one of these in your day/week/year. If you have time, take five minutes today to research or plan. Put it in your diary.

TOP TIP

Whether it's in the next week or in six months, choose a specific date for your activity and get it in the diary.

MICROGAIN 7.5

DANCE LIKE NO ONE'S WATCHING!

We can lift our moods and be active at the same time by taking this small, joyful step. Music and dance have been found to be uplifting, energizing mood-raisers. They can leave us feeling brighter, more inspired and happier. Music can connect with our emotions and memories to help us process how we are feeling. It can promote relaxation and sleep, reduce stress, help us manage pain and improve memory. Studies have shown that athletes can benefit from improved performance by using music as part of their training and preparation.[20] Dance has also been associated with positive mental health.

Take a moment to consider a song or piece of music that you know lifts you up and never fails to make you smile. This might be a current song, or a song from your childhood, teenage years, university days or adulthood. It may be a silly song, or a song that reminds you of your friends, of wild nights or close connections. It might be a song that makes you want to sing out loud, or perform a familiar routine. If you aren't sure what your song might be, pick a favourite radio station or playlist on a streaming service with a style or era of songs that you know you love, and then wait for the right melody to play.

Find your song and put it on – loudly, if you can. Let yourself sing, dance, move. Be as free, as silly and as joyful as you can.

GET YOUR GROOVE ON

You might consider:

- Songs that you know all the words to
- Songs you know the dance moves to
- Songs from your past that resonate with you
- Motivational songs, e.g., songs from movies

Sometimes, depending on our moods, music and dance can help us express more difficult emotions. When we are feeling sad, angry, agitated, sad or hopeless, we can choose music that reflects our emotions and allows us to feel them. For example, the right songs allow us to cry or shout out in anger, or connect with frustrated lyrics.

Bringing music and dance into your life could mean:

- Listening to music whilst doing housework
- Listening to music whilst exercising
- Listening to music whilst getting ready to go out/you're in the shower
- Putting music on for a kitchen disco
- Listening to music to hype you up before a big job interview
- Listening to music on your daily commute or walk
- Listening to music during your wind-down routine before bed

MICROGAIN CHALLENGE

Put a song on now, wherever you are, whatever you are doing.
Put headphones on, or blare it out from speakers or your phone. Bonus points if you can let yourself go and dance around the room.

If this isn't possible, consider taking a minute to write a list of your favourite songs, or do a quick poll of the people around you to find out which songs lift them up, and then pop one of their suggestions on.

Commit to bringing some music and dance into your life at some point today. Set yourself a reminder if you need.

TOP TIP

Make a playlist that lifts you up, makes you feel good and makes you smile, that you can easily turn on when you need a boost.

CHAPTER 8

MICROGAINS TO TAKE CARE OF YOUR EMOTIONS

"Emotions are like a river, constantly flowing and changing. They are like the weather, constantly moving and passing through. The storm gives way to sun, the sun may move behind the clouds..."

Dr Emma

"Feelings are something you have: not something you are."[21]

Shannon L Alder, life coach and writer

THE MICROGAINS

1. Understand Your Emotions
2. Notice and Name Your Feelings
3. Sit with Your Feelings
4. Self-Soothe
5. Express Emotions Healthily

As humans we are emotional beings. We feel many different emotions throughout our human experience. This emotional experience is deeply connected within our minds and bodies. We can experience an emotion as a feeling and also as a physical sensation through how our bodies change.

Emotions are processed through parts of the brain including the amygdala, and can be part of the nervous system's response to a threat. For example, we can feel anxiety, fear and anger (sympathetic nervous system activation) or calm and soothed (parasympathetic nervous system activation).

Learning to notice and name our emotions; understand, accept and make space for our emotions; respond kindly to ourselves when we experience emotions; and find helpful ways to manage our emotional responses are all incredibly psychologically healthy and helpful skills we can develop. These skills help us regulate our emotions more compassionately and effectively, and they often help us support others with their emotions too.

As you read through this section, it may make you reflect on how you think about emotions and how you see a place for them in your daily life. Often we are influenced by our lives and early childhood experiences as to whether we see emotions as positive and manageable or scary and negative. You might find yourself thinking that negative emotions aren't okay, or that you should try to shut them down, hide them, suppress them and not feel them. Or you might notice that you struggle to contain your emotions and they get too big and overwhelming for you and others. Or you might find you have already developed some of the skills we'll cover and feel quite confident in your emotional regulation.

However you come to this section, we hope you find these microgain ideas helpful as part of your overall journey toward better wellbeing and mental health.

Please note: If this section feels really tricky for you and you find managing emotions hard, then please do consider reaching out for therapy support.

MICROGAIN 8.1

UNDERSTAND YOUR EMOTIONS

To be human is to experience emotions. How we understand and manage our emotions is typically influenced by our early childhoods, and what we learnt about emotions and managing emotions from our caregivers, and through our life experiences – especially moments of big or painful emotions, such as during times of trauma, extreme stress, betrayal, grief and loss.

To help make sense of, feel and respond to our emotions in the most psychologically healthy ways, it can help to understand some shared principles about emotions. We want to share two key principles here:

1. To feel different emotions is to be human.
2. Emotions are like the weather.

TO FEEL DIFFERENT EMOTIONS IS TO BE HUMAN

It is normal and understandable for humans to experience a full range of emotions over the course of a day, week, month or lifetime. We are not designed to only feel the "good" or positive emotions. To be human is to feel everything – happiness, sadness, anger, satisfaction, regret, joy, excitement, shame, worry, love and so on.

Giving ourselves permission to feel all these emotions is important. Russ Harris, in his work within acceptance and commitment therapy (ACT) talks about the concept that even on your happiest day, you are likely to feel other emotions too – annoyance, stress, sadness that the day is over, etc. If we let ourselves accept that all emotions are normal, human and, ultimately, welcome, then we start from a place of peace where different emotions may be present. This is far more effective than expecting to only have the "positive" emotions.

EMOTIONS ARE LIKE THE WEATHER

"Emotions are like the weather" is another lovely concept/ metaphor used widely when describing emotions within general wellbeing writing and therapy approaches. The concept is based on the idea that we can consider our emotions to be like a weather system – constantly moving and changing.

In this metaphor we are the sky, the constant blue. And the emotions are the sunshine, the clouds, the rain, the wind, the storms, the bright, clear days and the grey, heavy fog. As with the weather, emotions constantly move and flow, sometimes within the same hour, certainly within the same day, week and month.

Understanding this concept enables us to know that whatever we may be experiencing, it will flow, move and change; no feeling stays static and constant, just as the weather doesn't. So knowing the storms will always pass is important. And understanding that even on a sunny day, we might get a cooler breeze – or a couple of grey clouds – before the sun comes out again is also important.

MICROGAIN CHALLENGE

Reflect on these two principles and how they make sense to you.

Reflect on how you can apply these to yourself and your experience of emotions.

TOP TIP

Reflect on your day and the metaphor of your emotions as the weather. How have your emotions moved and changed through today, even in small ways? What weather system would you compare each emotional experience to?

MICROGAIN 8.2

NOTICE AND NAME
YOUR FEELINGS

Part of being human means we may, at any given time, experience a whole range of emotions: happiness, sadness, anger, anxiety, guilt, shame, sadness, worry, fear, to name but a few.

Being able to NOTICE and NAME the feeling has been shown to have a positive effect on our ability to make sense of and manage the feeling. This might seem simple, yet it isn't always something we find easy or remember to do.

HOW TO NOTICE AND NAME

At any time in your day, try this exercise:

- Stop, pause, take a breath.
- Take a moment to notice how you are. Let any words come to mind.
- Now ask yourself, "How I am feeling right now?" Is there one word that best describes how you feel, or do you feel you are holding a few different feelings at once?
- If you can identify a feeling, is this just the tip of the iceberg? Are there any feelings underneath this one, below the surface? For example, you might be feeling stressed or angry, but are there any other emotions lurking underneath? Are you also holding sadness, disappointment, worry or fear?
- Let yourself just notice and name this for a moment. Say to yourself, "I am feeling X right now." Say it with compassion

for yourself, if this is a tough emotion. Or say it with pride or joy if this is a feeling you want to celebrate.

• Notice how it feels to acknowledge this emotion. What does it tell you about what you may need right now?

Please note: For anyone struggling to find words for their emotions, search online for "emotions wheel" or "feelings wheel" to find a very detailed colour wheel of many different words to describe emotions.

MICROGAIN CHALLENGE

Try this exercise right now. Experiment with finding the right words to describe how you feel.

TOP TIP

Use this exercise at different times of day. Try it when you are feeling calm or in a good place, and then when you are holding stress or a negative emotion of some kind.

MICROGAIN 8.3

SIT WITH YOUR FEELINGS

Current mental health guidance, especially for parents and children, emphasizes the importance of witnessing, sitting with and staying with our children during big emotions. This is likely still a work in progress for most parents; indeed, for most of us adults, this might be new learning.

As we grow up, it is not uncommon to learn habits and strategies that *shut down* emotions, push them away or minimize them. Yet we know that when we do this, psychologically, the emotion rarely disappears in a healthy way. As psychologist Carl Yung is commonly reported to have said, "What you resist, [...] persists."[22] And indeed, it often simmers under the surface, or bubbles over, spilling out where we least want it to.

These strategies to avoid or deny emotions also teach us that emotions are somehow bad, wrong, harmful or unmanageable. And this all stops us learning that if we can begin to notice and name our feelings (Microgain 8.2), and *stay with* our feelings – sitting with them, making space for them, turning toward them and allowing them to be present – we are able to manage them and move through them much more effectively.

This work is about healthy emotional regulation and expression, and not about giving our emotions free rein to become overwhelming, uncontained, unregulated, or distressing for us and everyone around us. If you do feel as though your emotions have taken over, try one of the grounding exercises from Microgains 2.3 and 2.4.

HOW TO STAY WITH AND SIT WITH AN EMOTION

When you notice a difficult or big emotion, see if you can allow it to be present and make space for it. Try just accepting it is there and breathing through it. This skill is about allowing yourself to feel it, rather than suppressing it or trying to get rid of it.

What we expect is that when we learn to do this, the emotion begins to feel more possible to feel, to tolerate, to cope with, and often it begins to gently subside.

Try these steps:

1. Take a deep breath.
2. Notice and name the emotion (Microgain 8.2).
3. Notice and name where you feel this in your body.
4. Take a deep breath and picture making space for the feeling in your mind and body.
5. With every breath imagine you are expanding the space around the feeling.
6. Give yourself permission to stay with the emotion for just a little longer than you might usually tolerate – noticing it, naming it, feeling it, without judgement. This might start with 10–30 seconds and build to one minute. (For BIG emotions you might combine this with the grounding exercise in Microgain 2.3.)
7. As you feel this emotion, send yourself love and compassion. (You could combine this with the kind hands exercise in Microgain 3.3.)
8. As time goes on and you practise this exercise, aim to be able to stay with the feeling and notice as it rises and falls, moving and passing through, enabling you to cope.

MICROGAIN CHALLENGE

If you are feeling a difficult emotion right now, practise this exercise.

If not, choose a recent situation that ignites difficult emotions when you think about it. (Aim for something that's no more than a 5 out of 10 in terms of emotional difficulty as you practise this.)

TOP TIP

As you take a breath, imagine the space around the feeling expanding, even by a little bit. Creating space helps you feel like you are able to contain this feeling.

MICROGAIN 8.4

SELF-SOOTHE

Finding healthy and effective ways to soothe ourselves when we have the inevitable difficult feelings that come with being human can be life-changing. These strategies enable us to feel well and function, whilst experiencing a full range of emotions.

Equally, identifying any problematic ways in which we may self-soothe is important too – we likely all recognize how using alcohol, drugs, food or sex to "calm" or soothe (or most likely numb) is rarely healthy or helpful for our functioning and wellbeing. If this is something you struggle with, we would encourage you to seek support for this, whether through self-help or professional support. It's beyond the scope of this book to fully address here.

Developing healthy ways to soothe our feelings means that when we feel a difficult, big or painful emotion, we have a toolkit of strategies to draw on that can help calm us as that feeling moves through us. It means that we have the ability to regulate our bodies' physiological response so that an emotion does not overwhelm us.

HOW TO SELF-SOOTHE

Here are small ways in which we can soothe ourselves during difficult or painful emotions:

1. Stop, pause, notice and name emotions (Microgain 8.2).
2. *Give yourself permission* to have any feeling, and accept that being human means experiencing the whole range of emotions at some point in time.

3. Use slow, deep breaths to calm your nervous system (Microgain 2.1).

4. Try the kind hands exercise (Microgain 3.3).

5. Cuddle or stroke a pet and allow yourself to feel calmed by the connection (Microgain 5.2).

6. Have a cuddle with a loved one.

7. Remind yourself that this *is* painful but it *will* ebb, flow and pass if you let it (Microgain 8.1).

8. Use calm and kind self-talk – use compassionate words, as well as AND (Microgain 3.5): "This is hard/painful AND I can get through this."

9. Use the dropping-anchor exercise (Microgain 2.3), or scent, ice or warmth (Microgain 2.4) to ground yourself.

10. Wrap your arms around yourself for a self-hug.

11. Remind yourself of what you have been through, so you might start to understand why this feeling has shown up (rather than criticizing yourself for having this feeling).

12. Hold a heating pad on your lap or in your arms.

13. Take a warm shower or bath.

14. Listen to soothing music.

15. Sit somewhere comfortable and wrap a blanket around yourself.

MICROGAIN CHALLENGE

Read through the list and see which strategy, or which three strategies, feels or would feel most helpful for you in times of difficult emotions.

Make a note of these strategies in your phone or diary to remind yourself.

TOP TIP

Remember, we soothe ourselves with compassion – this flows through all these strategies. See Chapter 3 for more support with this concept.

MICROGAIN 8.5

EXPRESS EMOTIONS HEALTHILY

We've been exploring ways to understand and make space for our emotions. At times it may be that noticing, naming, sitting with, and accepting and soothing ourselves is all we need. But it is also important to be able to express our emotions and communicate these to others in healthy ways.

We have explored the fact that we are social creatures who value connection – with ourselves and others. This can also be seen in the way we can regulate our emotions through expressing ourselves outwardly.

Of course, we can express our emotions in unhelpful or less-healthy ways. Sometimes our emotions can come out in angry behaviour – shouting, storming off. Sometimes they can come out in unkind comments or overwhelming distress, or through coping mechanisms, such as turning to food, drugs or alcohol. It may show up in "sulking" and withdrawal behaviours, or in pretending we are fine.

As well as building healthy ways of expressing emotions, it can also be important to reflect on any unhelpful ways we express our emotions that we might want to change in time.

HOW TO EXPRESS AND COMMUNICATE EMOTION IN HEALTHY OR HELPFUL WAYS

- Acknowledge to yourself what you are feeling, and allow yourself to compassionately consider *why* you may be feeling this. This includes letting yourself consider what you are going through in your life right now and what you may have gone through in your life previously. This can often help you have more insight into why you may be experiencing the emotions that you are. (If you find this tricky, imagine how you would support a friend with the same experiences and understand their emotions.) The idea of the "capacity cup" is also important here. If you are full to capacity with your different roles and everything you are carrying (stressors), then it is often far easier for emotions to spill out and feel big. Recognize if this is what is going on and be kind to yourself about this.

- Give yourself permission to feel, without criticism and judgement. Know that you can be struggling because you are human, but this doesn't make you bad, weak, a failure, or any of the other negative critiques your mind might make up.
- Share with a loved one about how you are feeling. Try to do this from a grounded space (see Microgain 2.3). Consider how they might be able to help, and let them know this – even just by asking them to listen or give you a hug.
- Let a manager or member of the occupational health team at work know if you are struggling. Consider what help you might need right now.
- Journal. Let yourself free-write how you are feeling, or focus on a specific aspect of the emotional experience or issue, to help you release and process what you are carrying.
- Listen to some music or a playlist that reflects how you are feeling. Try playing it loudly in the car.
- Read poems or writings that connect with the emotions you are experiencing. (For example, Donna Ashworth's poetry about life and loss can be a lovely place to start – see the Resources at the back of the book for more information.)
- Go for walk in nature and let yourself *just be* with your feelings.
- Access support and therapy. Source a qualified counsellor, psychotherapist, accredited therapist (e.g.,

in cognitive behavioural therapy (CBT) or eye movement desensitization and reprocessing (EMDR)), or clinical or counselling psychologist.

MICROGAIN CHALLENGE

Choose one strategy you would find helpful when you need to express an emotion.
Make a note of this so you can use it when you need.

TOP TIP

If you would find it helpful to talk to someone, make a note of the people you would feel comfortable to talk to, so you can easily do this when you need. Refer to your connection tree (Microgain 5.3) to remind yourself of your options.

CHAPTER 9

MICROGAINS FOR
HOW YOU THINK

"The mind loves telling stories; in fact, it never stops."[23]

Russ Harris, psychotherapist

THE MICROGAINS

1. Remember: Thoughts Aren't Facts
2. Notice Problematic Thinking
3. Problem-Solve a Worry
4. Let Go
5. Be Flexible

All day long our minds are full of thoughts. It has been suggested that we have 6,000 thoughts every single day. We think about ourselves, others, our current situations, possible future outcomes or past traumas. We have thoughts about what we hope or fear.

These thoughts flash through our minds every day, sometimes so fast we don't notice them or fully tune into them. Sometimes we notice how we *feel* first, and this then leads us to identify our thoughts. Sometimes we only notice our thinking when we stop and ask ourselves what we think about a situation. Other times our thoughts are constantly spiralling and whirling, competing for our attention.

Our thoughts are very powerful. They can help lift us up and drive us forward; they can also be very problematic. There is a close, interconnected relationship between our thoughts, emotions, physical feelings and behaviour. This highlights how powerful our thoughts are.

It is also important to learn that our thoughts can be biased, distorted, exaggerated and, at times, plain untrue. Understanding this and how to harness the power of our thoughts is an essential set of skills we can develop.

MICROGAIN 9.1

REMEMBER:
THOUGHTS AREN'T FACTS

The way we think has a significant impact on our mental wellbeing. Depending on how we think, we can feel happy, joyful, excited, anxious, angry, worried or scared. We can feel optimistic or hopeless. We can feel good about ourselves or terrible. This is the power our thoughts have. And yet, a very important principle that we often forget is that **the thoughts that go through our mind are not facts**.

Thoughts are perspectives, beliefs, judgements and opinions. They are influenced by our experiences, our moods, our belief systems, our fatigue levels, our personal biases and more. They are therefore not always evidence based, rational or based in reality. This doesn't mean there isn't factual information in our thoughts. But understanding that our thoughts are not factual is an important first step that can help us begin to manage them in a more effective way.

HOW TO REMIND YOURSELF THAT
THOUGHTS AREN'T FACTS

1. Identity a situation that is annoying you or creating some negative emotion.
2. What are you thinking about the situation, yourself, others, the past or the future?
3. Remind yourself that these thoughts are not facts. They are beliefs/perspectives/opinions.

4. Add in the phrase, "I am noticing I am having the thought that..." before the thought. This helps remind you this is just a thought, and creates some distance
5. Ask yourself: What is the evidence for this thought or these thoughts? If you were trying to prove them in a court of law, is there indisputable evidence?
6. Ask yourself: Do other people hold different beliefs or opinions about this situation? If there are multiple opinions, it is much more likely that your thought is a belief or assumption.
7. Ask yourself: Are there biases in these thoughts? Common biases include:
    - Catastrophizing – thinking the worst thing about a situation
    - Black-and-white thinking – thinking in "absolutes", e.g., all good or all bad
    - Comparing – comparing yourself unfavourably to others
    - Mind-reading – assuming you know what others are thinking about you
    - Emotional reasoning – assuming because you feel something, it must be true
    - Absolute statements – thoughts that include should, ought to, must, have to, etc.

MICROGAIN CHALLENGE

Think about a situation that has recently bothered you, or a time when you noticed your mood had changed.

Go through the steps above. Notice the difference in your experience of your thoughts when you consider what you are thinking is a *perspective* rather than a *fact*.

TOP TIP

See if you can notice which biases tend to creep into your thinking the most.

MICROGAIN 9.2

NOTICE PROBLEMATIC THINKING

THE STOPP METHOD

So far, we've established that we have thousands of thoughts a day; thoughts aren't facts; and our thoughts can stem from a mixture of factors – beliefs, perspectives and opinions – influenced by our past and present experiences, our worries, fears, hopes and wishes (Microgain 9.1).

So, given all this, what can we do with our thoughts? How can we help ourselves with our thinking? It can help to understand what is going on in our minds when we are thinking about a situation, and draw on some strategies to notice and think about the situation in more helpful ways. STOPP will help you do this.

USING "STOPP"

A lovely way to gain some perspective in relation to your thoughts is the STOPP exercise, a technique developed within the CBT approach.

This mindfulness-based exercise helps to create space between you and your thoughts, and can therefore help you to engage in more considered responses to your thinking.

S **Stop** and press pause where you are.

T **Take a breath**. Gently observe your breathing. Breathe in through your nose and out through your mouth. Try and slow your breathing down if you can. When we focus on our breathing, we are less focused on our difficult thoughts and feelings.

O **Observe**. Notice what thoughts are going through your mind at this moment. What are you paying attention to? What are you noticing in your body and your surroundings, as well as your mind?

P **Pull back**. Imagine you are pulling out of your situation – like zooming out on a map, or like a drone flying away from you and observing from a wider angle. Ask yourself:

- What does the bigger picture look like?
- How else could I look at the situation?
- What other perspectives are there? What is a more neutral perspective?
- How else could I think about it? What is a more compassionate perspective?
- Is it important right now? Will it be important next week, next year?
- What would trusted others say about what I am experiencing right now?
- What would I say to a loved one if they were experiencing this?
- Does it benefit me to listen to these thoughts or let them influence my behaviour?

Seeing a bigger picture can give us a new perspective, and this can lead to a reduction in distress.

P **Practise what works**. If you zoom out and hold on to the bigger picture or wider perspective, what action needs to be taken right now, if any? How can you respond in a helpful, compassionate way for yourself or others? Can you link your response to your values (Microgain 10.2) and the person you want to be? Can you respond carefully, thoughtfully and compassionately rather than being impulsively or emotionally driven?

MICROGAIN CHALLENGE

Start slowly with this strategy. Focus on the first two steps and try to use them several times a day.

Try saying "STOPP" aloud to yourself during these moments. Start with less-distressing thoughts and work up to using the exercise for more distressing ones when you are ready.

TOP TIP

Slowly try adding in an extra step when you feel confident with the previous one. As you move forward, run through all the steps at least 5–6 times each day.

MICROGAIN 9.3

PROBLEM-SOLVE A WORRY

We all have worries, issues on our minds, unresolved problems we might be dwelling on.

Are you a worrier? Do you have many worries, or just a few that show up now and again? Can you identify a worry right now that has been bothering you?

Worries can swirl around in our minds, causing us to ruminate or spiral from one worry to another, escalating without us even realizing it. When we are full of worry, this can, of course, leave us feeling anxious, on edge, preoccupied or scared. It can make it hard to focus, and it can be physically exhausting to have worries in our minds.

Whilst feeling worried is part of the human experience, for some people this can become too frequent and all encompassing. Others may find themselves really stuck with certain worries during stressful periods of life.

The main challenge with worry is when we let it fester without addressing it. We can get stuck in that worry and not ever take action to resolve it. Sometimes this happens because we aren't thinking past the worry itself; sometimes this is because we hadn't considered problem-solving or had any sense that we could resolve it; sometimes it's because we may feel anxious about addressing it. And yet, of course, problem-solving a worry head-on can often help us resolve it and free us from the cycle of worry.

PROBLEM-SOLVING EXERCISE

Instead of staying *in* the worry, try this quick exercise:

1. Identify a worry – write it down. *I am worried about...* You might want to choose a small worry to start with.
2. If it is unclear after step 1, ask yourself what specifically it is that you are worried about happening.
3. Now ask: Is there anything I can do about this worry? Is there any practical action I can take? (Please note: Sometimes there are worries we can do nothing about, and sometimes there are practical things we can do to address a worry.)
4. If there is nothing you can do about the worry, make a commitment to set it down and let it go because worrying about something you can do nothing about isn't helpful or effective.
5. If there is something you *can* do, problem-solve what this is, when you can do it and how you can do it. Make this plan as specific as possible. And take that action.

MICROGAIN CHALLENGE

Work through the five steps, problem-solving a worry you are holding now.
Repeat this as many times as necessary for new worries.

TOP TIP

Once you have problem-solved a worry and made a plan, write this down and come back to it whenever you need to remind yourself of the process.

MICROGAIN 9.4

LET GO

How often do you find yourself stuck on an issue? How often do you find yourself going over a conversation or an interaction that has happened? How often do you find yourself mentally holding on to something, finding it hard to let go or move on? How does it feel having this consume your mind, even when the situation has long passed or may never happen?

If your answer to the above questions is "quite often", then these next steps might work for you. Finding a way to let things go can bring you peace and calm. It can reduce your stress and enable you to move forward, without harbouring these ongoing issues in your mind.

STEPS TO LET GO

1. Acknowledge what the issue is and that you are ready to let it go. Make sure you have problem-solved (Microgain 9.3) or sought help for the issue (Microgain 7.3) first. Choosing to let go might also be part of your process of cultivating a more positive mindset (Microgain 10.4) or practising self-compassion (Microgain 3.1).
2. Acknowledge what it is costing you to keep holding on to this issue.
3. Apply the workability concept, developed by Russ Harris (see the Resources section for more information). Ask yourself: Does it help me? Does it benefit me if I continue thinking/ ruminating on this, or would it be more helpful to set it down and let it go?

4. Give yourself *permission* to let go. Make the decision to set something down and reduce ruminating on it.
5. Practise mindfulness (Microgain 1.1) to gently notice as the issue pops into your mind. Allow it to float in and out, without getting dragged into spiralling/ruminating on the issue.
6. Imagine letting the thoughts go – like leaves dropping onto a stream and floating away.
7. Imagine you are in a tug-of-war with your thoughts. Picture dropping the rope and not holding on to the thoughts any more.
8. Practise redirecting your mind to another task or activity.

Practise any/all of the above as needed – be aware that persistent thoughts might keep popping back in your mind, so you may need to repeat these steps numerous times. That is completely normal.

MICROGAIN CHALLENGE

Consider an issue or thought (start small to begin with) and make a choice to let go.

Practise the steps above. How does this feel? Can you keep practising?

TOP TIP

Expand the imagery of letting thoughts go. Imagine them floating into the air on a balloon and drifting away. You might have to keep "releasing balloons" if the thoughts pop back.

MICROGAIN 9.5

BE FLEXIBLE

Psychological flexibility is a very useful and healthy skill to develop and one that will benefit you every single day.

Psychological flexibility refers to our ability to bend our thinking, our approaches, our perspectives and our reflections. It's our ability to listen, learn and incorporate new information. It's our ability to consider a new way of thinking or a new path of behaviour, and our ability to adapt to change.

Being flexible can work well when we connect to our values (Microgain 10.2) and use these to steer our choices as each day progresses, even if the content or plan for that day has to change (often due to circumstances outside our control).

Being flexible means being able to stay in touch with how we are doing at any moment in time so that we can then adjust and adapt to what we want and need.

These quotes capture the essence of this process:

"Stay committed to your decisions, but stay flexible in your approach." [24]

Tony Robbins, author, coach and speaker

"Flexibility requires an open mind and a welcoming of new alternatives." [25]

Deborah Day, mental health clinician and author

"Freedom and happiness are found in the flexibility and ease with which we move through change." [26]

Gautama Buddha, monk and spiritual teacher

"Psychological flexibility is the ability to feel and think with openness, to attend voluntarily to your experience of the present moment, and to move your life in directions that are important to you, building habits that allow you to live life in accordance with your values and aspirations."[27]

Steven C Hayes, psychology professor,
author and therapist; co-founder of
Acceptance and Commitment Therapy

WHAT PSYCHOLOGICAL FLEXIBILITY CAN LOOK LIKE

- Being mindful in the moment to new information/activities/ pathways and responding to them
- Being able to zoom out, in any situation, and look at the bigger picture
- Being able to ask, "What has happened to me?" or "What have I been through?" rather than, "What is wrong with me?"
- Being open to incorporate new information into your thinking
- Being able to consider that your thoughts are not facts (Microgain 9.1)
- Being open to update/adapt your conclusion on a topic when new information becomes available
- Being able to change your plans to respond to your needs (e.g., taking a break or going to bed early, working more or less, exercising, eating, drinking, etc.)
- Being able to revise your day if things don't go to plan

MICROGAIN CHALLENGE

Consider one way that being flexible in your thoughts may improve a situation for you today.

TOP TIP

Consider flexibility as a strength, enabling you to move with any situation, flowing and adapting as needed.

CHAPTER 10

MICROGAINS ABOUT YOU

"Time spent on you will always be valuable."

Dr Emma

THE MICROGAINS

1. Meet Your Needs
2. Connect with Your Values
3. Journal Five Good Things
4. Create Little Moments
5. Cultivate a Positive Mindset

Throughout this book we have written about ways to take care of your mental health. Each section has focused on a different area: mindfulness, being active, social connection, and so on.

In this section the focus is purely on you. On meeting your needs, connecting with yourself, taking care of yourself. Taking the time and energy to invest in you, in your wellbeing and your mental health, is what this book is all about, and will always be valuable.

We hope these five microgains inspire you to take extra steps to take care of you today.

MICROGAIN 10.1

MEET YOUR NEEDS

The message of this microgain might feel really simple: Don't forget to meet your basic needs.

Perhaps it seems pretty straightforward. Yet actually it's really easy to neglect your basic needs. How often have you sat at your desk, feeling hungry or thirsty, but not got up to meet this need? How often have you felt exhausted but not gone to bed early? How often have you wanted or needed a break but not taken one? Or been too hot/too cold without taking action to cool down/warm up? Or sat with a pain, headache or body stiffness longer than you needed to? We imagine you've been able to see yourself in at least one of these. With that, you can see how it's actually surprisingly easy to neglect your basic needs without even realizing.

So this microgain is a simple reminder to nudge you back toward taking care of yourself and your needs. And why is this important? Because these are often the basic pillars we need to feel and function well in ourselves, both mentally and physically. Consider prioritizing:

- Water/hydration
- Food/fuel
- Rest and sleep
- Maintaining temperature
- Managing your body pain/aches
- Taking care of yourself if you're unwell

CHECK IN TO MEET YOUR NEEDS

Take a moment for yourself and consider the following questions:

- Are you thirsty? Have you had enough water today – and if not, can you get yourself some now?
- Are you hungry? Do you need fuel or sustenance – and if so, can you action this now?
- Do you need a break or to prioritize rest? Can you do this now or plan this as soon as possible?
- Have you had enough sleep? Do you need to go to bed early or take steps to improve sleep (Microgain 4.3)?
- Are you warm/cold? Can you adjust the temperature for yourself now?
- Are you experiencing body aches/stiffness/pain? Do you need to look at pain management? Do you need to get up and move your body around, do some stretches or change position (Microgain 6.1)?
- Are you unwell? Do you need to rest, take a day off, see a doctor?

MICROGAIN CHALLENGE

Are you neglecting one of your basic needs?

Review at least one basic need and take steps to meet it if/as needed. Choose one need to take action on right now. How does it feel to meet these promptly through your day?

TOP TIP

If you know you routinely neglect these needs, make a note on your phone/diary, or pop a Post-it note on your laptop, to remind you to check in on your needs more regularly.

MICROGAIN 10.2

CONNECT WITH YOUR VALUES

A really useful method to help us navigate life is to focus on our values.

Many of us live our lives by the goals we set, from everyday goals to longer-term, larger goals. These can be great – they drive us forward and give us something to aim for. But it can also be tricky if we don't attain them. We can become deflated and think negatively about ourselves and our abilities. Whilst there will always be a place for goal setting and goal-focused behaviours, another way we can guide ourselves forward in life is by focusing on our *values* instead.

Values underlie everything we do – including our goals. In fact, our values are often described as a compass that helps navigate us toward what is important to us. They help us connect to what is important and meaningful to us; to what really matters deep down; and to the people we want to be, how we want to behave and the way we want to live, interact with others and take care of ourselves.

The good thing about values is that we can always find a way to live by them, even when our goals become difficult or impossible to achieve. Plus, knowing our values helps inform the types of goals we want to make and keep focused on. And if, during difficult moments, you are still able to connect with your values and what matters to you, this can help you navigate these tough times.

FIND YOUR VALUES

So, values are the compass that help guide how you live your life and who you want to be. Some examples of common values are:

Adventure	Kindness	Courage	Honesty
Love	Fitness	Justice	Fun
Connection	Persistence	Assertiveness	Compassion
Authenticity	Self-awareness	Health	Excitement

When working out your values:

- Read through a list of common values (above or find lists online).
- Instinctively and/or with reflection, as feels right, identify which values mean the most to you. You'll likely think most of them look good, but which ones *really* connect with who you are and how you want to live your life?
- See if you can pick your top three values that represent something important about who you are and how you want to live.
- Reflect on why these values matter to you.
- Reflect on how you can live your life with these values as your compass. Would you make any changes?

MICROGAIN CHALLENGE

Identify one value that really means something to you.

With this value in mind, reflect on the person you want to be and how you want to live your life.

Now think about what it actually means to live your life today according to that value. How would you act? How would you connect with others? How would you engage with the tasks of the day? How can living your life by this value enrich your life today?

See if you can take at least one step today, guided by the value you have identified. How does this feel?

TOP TIP

Don't overthink it – you'll instinctively know which values feel right for you and connect with you.

MICROGAIN 10.3

JOURNAL FIVE GOOD THINGS

Journaling is an amazing and easily accessible activity – all we need is paper, a pen and a few minutes of your time. It's a great way to help make sense of our thoughts and emotions. It can help to get our thoughts out of our heads and onto paper. It can also create a degree of separation between ourselves and what we are experiencing, therefore allowing us to better understand ourselves and our experiences. Journaling is frequently recommended in therapy and as a wellbeing and mental health practice.

Journaling involves taking some time to write down thoughts and feelings, experiences and self-reflections. It involves being open and curious about what we are experiencing and moving away from judgement or self-criticism. It can free writing or structured around a particular focus or issue. It can be done daily, weekly or sporadically when you feel the need. There are no hard-and-fast rules, and there are many types of journaling to try – experiment to find one that works for you.

LEARNING TO JOURNAL

What will you use as your journal?

There are many journal formats and tailor-made mental health journals on the market. However, it is important to note that you don't need to acquire one of these in order to benefit from journaling. A piece of paper or basic notebook and a pen is all you need.

Whilst there are benefits of writing by hand for emotional health, you can also choose to journal using a digital platform. There are journaling apps and tutorials available to help with this, or you can use your preferred word processor for journaling on your computer.

When should you journal?
Creating a regular journaling habit has the best effect on wellbeing. Therefore, our advice is to schedule time each day to write in your journal.

Decide on a time of day that works well for you. There isn't a right or wrong time – just try to choose one and stick with it each day, as this will help journaling become part of your routine.

If this feels too much of a commitment right now, and writing on an ad hoc basis works for you, this is fine! Don't let structure be a barrier!

Free writing
To "free write" is to just let yourself journal about what is going on with you or what is on your mind in that moment.

Let yourself write. Write about your thoughts, your feelings, what you are experiencing, how it impacts on you. Write whatever you want to say – let it all out. As you get toward the end of the journaling session, you may want to ask yourself what you need right now or where you want to be able to go next, based on what you have been reflecting on.

Structured journaling
If you wish to use structure in your journaling, you may consider any or all of the following prompts, or you can find a whole range of journaling prompts on the internet if you want to explore this further. Try writing about:

- What you are grateful for
- What you are proud of
- Your future hopes or aspirations
- Your progress today
- Your goals and how you want to connect with these, why they matter and how you can move toward them
- Values – what matters to you deep in your heart and how you want to live each day
- Your challenges and how you plan to overcome these

Always journal with compassion and care, acknowledging how you are doing and how you can best take care of yourself.

FIVE GOOD THINGS ABOUT YOU

Try this structured journal practice. Take five minutes to write and reflect on:

1. One thing you are grateful for
2. One thing you like about yourself
3. One thing you are hopeful for
4. One thing you want to work toward
5. One thing you value

MICROGAIN CHALLENGE

Try the Five Good Things journal practice for five minutes each day for a week.

Read back what you have written each day, and notice how you think and feel about what you have written.

TOP TIP

Start small. Before you start writing, take a few moments to reflect on how you are in that moment. Take a breath. Do you notice anything in the way your body feels or the emotions you're experiencing that you can take into your journaling?

MICROGAIN 10.4

CREATE LITTLE MOMENTS

DO SOMETHING NICE FOR YOURSELF

Taking care of your mental health includes believing you deserve to do nice things for yourself. Through small actions you can show yourself compassion and give yourself permission to experience lovely moments. Even in the midst of difficult times, it is always possible to give yourself little pockets of joy, peace, calm, happiness, love and care.

As we know, it is easy for our minds to be critical or negative toward us. Anything we can do to add kindness, understanding and compassion to our lives is positive for our wellbeing. Any action that communicates to yourself that you matter, you are important, you are worth caring for, you deserve good moments, you are valuable – is important. As with the impact of positive affirmations (Microgain 3.1), taking small actions to value yourself through the day can create an ongoing ripple effect so that you are more likely to value and take care of yourself.

Following on from the premise of Microgain 10.1, how often do you put your overall needs last, or even notice what your needs, wants or wishes are? How often does work, school, parenting or socializing come above your needs? How often do you prioritize doing something nice *just for you*?

Imagine what your day and life would be like if doing nice things for you – taking care of you – was just as important as taking care of or putting your energies into other things. A misconception widely held is that prioritizing yourself is to the detriment to other things.

INSPIRATION FOR CREATING A LITTLE MOMENT

Check out some ideas below, and see how they can add to your life, not take away from other parts of it.

- Buy yourself flowers.
- Make time to read a favourite book or some poetry.
- Take time to prepare a special coffee.
- Use a shower radio and play your favourite song in the shower.
- Walk your favourite route to work/school.
- Apply your moisturizer slowly as if you were having a facial.
- Choose your favourite meal for dinner.
- Give yourself the evening off – or a morning lie-in, guilt free.
- Go to bed early when you need.
- Give yourself a proper lunch break.
- Take time for self-pleasure.
- Listen to music or a podcast that makes you smile.
- Take a break and go for a walk.
- Book something nice – a massage, pamper appointment, time with friends.

MICROGAIN CHALLENGE

Choose one of the above, or come up with your own little moment. Do this for yourself now, or commit to doing this today.

TOP TIP

Aim to create at least one little moment for yourself every day.

MICROGAIN 10.5

CULTIVATE A POSITIVE MINDSET

Cultivating a positive mindset does not mean pretending everything is positive. It is also not getting drawn into "toxic positivity", which means you fail to acknowledge negative emotions, or dismiss others' anger or sadness and suggest they experience a positive feeling instead. It doesn't mean ignoring challenges. And it doesn't mean ignoring or invalidating any emotions you may be feeling (Microgain 8.3).

Cultivating a positive mindset means, when possible and appropriate, choosing a mindset that encourages a more optimistic, positive, hopeful outlook, one that veers more toward glass-half-full thinking and looks for solutions over barriers. This enables us to connect with and be more open to the range of positive emotions – happiness, contentment, peace, calm and joy.

HOW TO CREATE A POSITIVE MINDSET

Some ways to cultivate a positive mindset can include:

- Acknowledging challenges whilst being able to consider options to move forward
- Focusing on what you *can* do rather than becoming stuck on what you *can't*
- Identifying the strengths and skills you can bring to the situation
- Problem-solving solutions and options to overcome barriers
- Recognizing and acknowledging emotions, and accepting the reality of a situation in order to move forward – for example, you might acknowledge your frustration or sadness about not

having time to visit a loved one in your schedule, and then move gently toward acceptance of the situation, rather than just staying stuck in the feeling

- Considering how you might look at this through a positive or negative lens and see if it is more helpful to choose the positive
- Being open to finding the funny, the silly, the humour, the ridiculous in the situation in which you find yourself
- Considering how to make the best of a situation
- Practising talking to yourself with "can do" phrases and words of encouragement – "I can do this"; "We can figure this out"; "Let's find a way"
- Being open to flexible thinking (Microgain 9.5)
- Being open to finding moments of joy, gratitude and fun, even in hard times
- Picking a positive mantra or affirmation with which you can start your day (Microgain 3.2)

MICROGAIN CHALLENGE

Reflect on your typical mindset – do you naturally fall more toward a positive or negative mindset? Or somewhere in the middle?

Consider the strategies above and choose one you'd like to incorporate more. Think about a situation that is challenging right now and consider how cultivating a positive mindset may help you.

TOP TIP

Make a note in your phone/diary or journal of the strategy you want to try more. Try this for a situation that is only mildly challenging and keep practising.

FINAL WORDS

So there are your 50 microgains to improve your wellbeing and mental health. We hope you found them useful, inspiring and motivating. We hope you can choose your favourites and begin to incorporate them into your daily practice – and then be open to dipping back into this book at any time as you expand your practice.

Remember that these small moments count. Remember that, in line with the concept of marginal gains, if you take all of these small moments in your day, add in a mental health microgain and improve each of those moments by just 1%, you are going to have a significant overall increase in wellbeing and mental health. To build these habits we would encourage you to consider these ideas:

- Choose one microgain that you love and find a specific way to embed this into your life every day. It may help to connect it to something you are already doing daily (such as brushing your teeth – and then repeating your affirmations) to make it as easy as possible to add it in.
- Do this for one week, then choose your next microgain and begin to add this in, with the same principles as above. And then your next, and your next. Take your time to find what you love and what works for you, and be open to giving everything a try.
- Remember to be compassionate to yourself as you navigate your microgains. It can take time to master and build upon the skills we've introduced in this book.

If you want to learn more about the ideas and concepts explored here, dive into the resources section that follows.

A final prompt is to ask yourself each day: "What *one small thing* could I do today to take care of myself and enhance my wellbeing or mental health?" Maybe it is something from this book; maybe it is something else. Do it today.

For now, thank you for reading this book, for being open to learning and being inspired to find ways to look after yourself, live well and thrive.

Dr Emma and Dr Tara

INDEX OF MICROGAINS

1 MINDFUL MICROGAINS

2 MICROGAINS FOR BREATHING AND GROUNDING

3 COMPASSIONATE MICROGAINS

4 MICROGAINS TO REST AND SLEEP WELL

5 SOCIAL CONNECTION MICROGAINS

6 MOVEMENT MICROGAINS

7 PURPOSEFUL ACTION MICROGAINS

8 MICROGAINS TO TAKE CARE OF YOUR EMOTIONS

9 MICROGAINS FOR HOW YOU THINK

10 MICROGAINS ABOUT YOU

USEFUL RESOURCES

Here are some of our favourite books and podcasts that offer support for wellbeing and mental health.

BOOKS

Ashworth, Donna, *Loss* (2022), *I Wish I Knew* (2022), *Life* (2022), *Love* (2022), *Wild Hope* (2023), Black and White Publishing

Chatterjee, Dr Rangan, *The 4 Pillar Plan*, Penguin Life 2018

Clear, James, *Atomic Habits*, Random House Business 2018

Cotterill, Emma, *Your Mental Health Toolkit: A Card Deck*, Welbeck 2023

Ferguson, Anna, *The Vagus Nerve Reset*, Vermilion 2023

Greenberger, Dennis & Padesky, Christine, *Mind Over Mood*, Guilford Press 2015

Novogratz, Sukey & Novogratz, Elizabeth, *Just Sit*, Harper 2018

Quinn-Cirillo, Dr Tara & Trent, Dr Marianne, *Talking Heads: Your Guide to Finding a Qualified Therapist in the UK*, Independently published 2024

Reading, Suzy, *Rest to Reset* (2023), *Sit to Get Fit* (2023), Aster

Roslin, Gaby, *Spread the Joy*, HQ 2023

Sandeman, Stuart, *Breathe In Breath Out*, HQ 2022

Through this book we have drawn on concepts from therapy approaches such as Acceptance and Commitment Therapy, Cognitive Behavioural Therapy, Compassion Focused Therapy and trauma-informed approaches. Here are some books for further reading in this area:

Allan, Rachel, *How to Help Someone with Anxiety*, Welbeck 2021
Cotterill, Emma, *How to Help Someone with Depression*, Welbeck 2021
Harris, Russ, *ACT with Love*, New Harbinger 2023
Harris, Russ, *The Happiness Trap*, Robinson 2022
Hayes, Steven, A *Liberated Mind*, Vermilion 2019
Irons, Chris & Beaumont, Elaine, *The Compassionate Mind Workbook*, Robinson 2017
Neff, Kristin, *Self-Compassion*, Yellow Kite 2011
Smith, Julie, *Why Has Nobody Told Me This Before?*, Michael Joseph 2022
The *Overcoming* series from Robinson

PODCASTS

There are many brilliant podcasts out there. Here are just a few you might enjoy:

The Adversity Psychologist – Dr Tara Quinn-Cirillo
Feel Better Live More – Dr Rangan Chatterjee
Happy Place – Fearne Cotton
High Performance – Jake Humphrey and Damian Hughes
How to Fail – Elizabeth Day
Huberman Lab Podcast – Dr Andrew Huberman
The Insight Podcast – Samuel CW Hart
Just One Thing – Dr Michael Mosley
Ten Percent Happier – Dan Harris
We Can Do Hard Things – Glennon Doyle
Self Care Club – Lauren Mishcon and Nicole Goodman

ACKNOWLEDGEMENTS

Emma:

Writing this book has been a pleasure. To my co-author, Tara – thank you for your time, wisdom, enthusiasm and hard work!

Thank you to our wonderful editor, Beth, for your ongoing support.

Thank you to my friends and family for your love and encouragement, and to all the wonderful people I work with who inspire me every day.

And, of course, thank you always to my beautiful boys.

Tara:

My co-author and friend, Emma – we've known each other a long time, and it's been a pleasure to be able to write together! Thank you for teaching me so much.

Mum and Dad, my two amazing boys and niece Amy – thank you for your never-ending support. I love you to the moon and back!

Shirley, Marianne, Michaela – thanks for encouraging and holding space for me every day.

Heather and Julian, love you guys, and thanks for always helping me develop and remember my theoretical roots.

To Andy, thanks for being my constant motivator and also my "still". You help me see what's possible.

To our editors, Beth and Andrea – thanks for having me on board and teaching me so much!

REFERENCES

1   Allen, Eddie. (11 April 2024). Sir Dave Brailsford at British
    Cycling - A career retrospective. Available at: https://www.
    britishcycling.org.uk/gbcyclingteam/article/gbr20140411-
    British-Cycling---The-Brailsford-years-0
2   Harris, Russ. (2011). *The Reality Slap*. Little, Brown.
3   NHS. (n.d.) How to meditate for beginners. Available at:
    https://www.nhs.uk/every-mind-matters/mental-wellbeing-tips/
    how-to-meditate-for-beginners
4   John Hopkins Medicine. (n.d.). Breathing Techniques. https://
    www.hopkinsmedicine.org/breathlessness-clinic/breathing-
    techniques
5   Thích Nhất Hạnh. (1997). *Stepping into Freedom: An
    Introduction to Buddhist Monastic Training*. Parallax Press.
6   Sikuza, Judy. (13 May 2024). Thought leadership: Empowering
    the next generation of Mandelas. Available at: https://www.
    mandelarhodes.org/news-impact/news/thought-leadership-
    empowering-the-next-generation-of-mandelas
7   Neff, Kristin. (n.d.). What is Self-Compassion? Available at:
    https://self-compassion.org/what-is-self-compassion/#what-is-
    self-compassion
8   Neff, Kristin. (n.d.) Exercise 2: Self-Compassion Break. Available
    at: https://self-compassion.org/exercises/exercise-2-self-
    compassion-break/
9   Sri Sri Ravi Shankar. (2001). *Celebrating Silence*. Art of Living
    Foundation.

10 Dekker, Thomas. Quotable Quotes. Available at: https://www.
    goodreads.com/quotes/135448-do-but-consider-what-an-
    excellent-thing-sleep-is-that-golden
11 Dalton-Smith, Shaundra. (2018). *Sacred Rest*. FaithWords.
12 Bryan, Lucy, and Singh, Abhinav. (7 May 2024). Alcohol and
    Sleep. Available at: https://www.sleepfoundation.org/nutrition/
    alcohol-and-sleep
13 Pacheco, Danielle, and Cotilar, Dustin. (17 April 2024). Caffeine
    and Sleep. Available at: https://www.sleepfoundation.org/
    nutrition/caffeine-and-sleep
14 Brown, Brené. (2012). *Daring Greatly*. Avery.
15 Aked, Jody, Marks, Nic, Cordon, Corrina, and Thompson,
    Sam. (22 October 2008). Five Ways to Wellbeing. Available
    at: https://neweconomics.org/uploads/files/five-ways-to-
    wellbeing-1.pdf
16 Holmes, Tori. (n.d.) Can Dogs Sense Human Emotions?
    Available at: https://www.freshpet.com/en-gb/blog/can-dogs-
    sense-human-emotions
17 Needell, Nancy, and Mehta-Naik, Nisha. (December 2016). Is
    Pet Ownership Helpful in Reducing the Risk and Severity of
    Geriatric Depression? *Geriatrics (Basel)*, 1(4): 24. Available at:
    https://www.ncbi.nlm.nih.gov/pmc/articles/PMC6371194
18 Caron, Leslie. QuoteFancy. Available at: https://quotefancy.
    com/quote/1122800/Leslie-Caron-The-most-important-thing-is-
    to-remain-active-and-to-love-what-you-are-doing
19 Koyenikan, Idowu. (January 2016). *Wealth for All*. Grandeur
    Touch, LLC.
20 Martin, Deveon. (28 November 2023). The Pros and Cons of
    Listening to Music While Working Out. Available at: https://
    www.nifs.org/blog/the-pros-and-cons-of-listening-to-music-
    while-working-out
21 Alder, Shannon. (n.d.) Goodreads. Available at: https://www.
    goodreads.com/quotes/906515-feelings-are-something-you-
    have-not-something-you-are

REFERENCES

22 Seltzer, Leon. (15 June 2016). *You Only Get More of What You Resist—Why?* Available at: https://www.psychologytoday.com/gb/blog/evolution-the-self/201606/you-only-get-more-what-you-resist-why

23 Harris, Russ. (2022). *The Happiness Trap*. Robinson.

24 Robbins, Tony. (n.d.). Tony's Advice. Available at: www.tonyrobbins.com/ask-tony

25 Day, Deborah. (n.d.). Goodreads. Available at: https://www.goodreads.com/author/quotes/1438286.Deborah_Day

26 Siddartha Gautama. (n.d.). Goodreads. Available at: https://www.goodreads.com/quotes/846414-in-life-we-cannot-avoid-change-we-cannot-avoid-loss.

27 Hayes, Steven. (2019). *A Liberated Mind*. Vermillion.

TRIGGERHUB IS ONE OF THE MOST ELITE AND SCIENTIFICALLY PROVEN FORMS OF MENTAL HEALTH INTERVENTION

Trigger Publishing is the leading independent mental health and wellbeing publisher in the UK and US. Our collection of bibliotherapeutic books and the power of lived experience change lives forever. Our courageous authors' lived experiences and the power of their stories are scientifically endorsed by independent federal, state and privately funded research in the US. These stories are intrinsic elements in reducing stigma, making those with poor mental health feel less alone, giving them the privacy they need to heal, ensuring they are guided by the essential steps to kick-start their own journeys to recovery, and providing hope and inspiration when they need it most.

Clinical and scientific research conducted by assistant professor Dr Kristin Kosyluk and her highly acclaimed team in the Department of Mental Health Law & Policy at the University of South Florida (USF), as well as complementary research by her peers across the US, has independently verified the power of lived experience as a core component in achieving mental health prosperity. Their findings categorically confirm lived experience as a leading method in treating those struggling with poor mental health by significantly reducing stigma and the time it takes for them to seek help, self-help or signposting if they are struggling.

Delivered through TriggerHub, our unique online portal and smartphone app, we make our library of bibliotherapeutic titles and other vital resources accessible to individuals and organizations anywhere, at any time and with complete privacy, a crucial element of recovery. As such, TriggerHub is the primary recommendation across the UK and US for the delivery of lived experiences.

At Trigger Publishing and TriggerHub, we proudly lead the way in making the unseen become seen. We are dedicated to humanizing mental health, breaking stigma and challenging outdated societal values to create real action and impact. Find out more about our world-leading work with lived experience and bibliotherapy via triggerhub.com, or by joining us on:

- 🐦 @triggerhub_
- 🅕 @triggerhub.org
- 📷 @triggerhub_

Dr Kristin Kosyluk, PhD, is an assistant professor in the Department of Mental Health Law & Policy at USF, a faculty affiliate of the Louis de la Parte Florida Mental Health Institute, and director of the STigma Action Research (STAR) Lab. Find out more about Dr Kristin Kosyluk, her team and their work by visiting:

USF Department of Mental Health Law & Policy:
www.usf.edu/cbcs/mhlp/index.aspx

USF College of Behavioral and Community Sciences:
www.usf.edu/cbcs/index.aspx

STAR Lab: www.usf.edu/cbcs/mhlp/centers/star-lab/

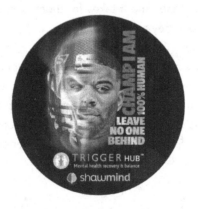

For more information, visit BJ-Super7.com